The Meaning of Illness

Social Orders
A series of monographs and tracts
Edited by Jacques Revel and Marc Augé
Ecole des Hautes Etudes en Sciences Sociales, Paris, France

This book is part of a series. The publisher will accept continuation orders which may be
cancelled at any time and which provide for the automatic billing and shipping of each title
in the series upon publication. Please write for details.

The Meaning of Illness
Anthropology, History and Sociology

Edited by

Marc Augé and *Claudine Herzlich*

Translated from the French

by

Katherine J. Durnin
Caroline Lambein
Karen Leclercq-Jones
Barbara Puffer Garnier
and Ronald W. Williams

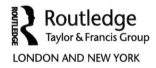

Routledge
Taylor & Francis Group
LONDON AND NEW YORK

First published 1995 by Routledge

2 Park Square, Milton Park, Abingdon, Oxon OX14 4RN
711 Third Avenue, New York, NY 10017, USA

Routledge is an imprint of the Taylor & Francis Group, an informa business

First issued in paperback 2016

Transferred to Digital Printing 2011

British Library Cataloguing in Publication Data

Meaning of Illness: Anthropology, History
and Sociology – (Social Order Series, ISSN 0275–7524, Vol. 5)
  I. Augé, Marc II. Herzlich, Claudine
  III. Durnin, Katherine J. IV. Series
  306-461

  ISBN 978-3-7186-5207-5 (hbk)
  ISBN 978-1-138-98063-1 (pbk)

Publisher's Note
The publisher has gone to great lengths to ensure the quality of this reprint but points out that some imperfections in the original may be apparent.

CONTENTS

SOCIAL ORDERS

The social sciences propose a renewed understanding of the contemporary world. In social matters they endeavour to draw attention to orders, relationships, levels of organization which, at the same time, define systems of intelligibility. They do not do so peremptorily but strive to construct them gradually, by approximations and by trial and error. To understand the social orders, the social sciences mobilize the knowledge and the practices peculiar to various fields of interest irrespective of the divisions between disciplines: the anthropologist, the historian, the economist and the sociologist gather together here around objects which have been constructed in common. It is this laboratory work that the **SOCIAL ORDERS** collection wishes to present in this account of the current state of our on-going research.

FOREWORD

This book is based on a collection of essays written in the early 1980s in which a group of researchers demonstrated a shift away from how the social sciences were at that time strictly divided into their respective disciplines regarding the analyses of societies, each of which had been too closely designated by a particular field of research. The overlap between anthropology, sociology and history, and African societies' fluctuating relationship with industrialized societies are the two indiscernible elements that characterize our research in this work.

This book has been published in English more than ten years later. Since then, radical change has occurred, both in the social sciences and in society. The outbreak of AIDS in Africa as well as in the industrialized countries does not represent the least of the radical change; this societal trauma alone would suffice for the basis of the application of the new cross disciplinary approach used in this book. Although today's reader will probably notice the time that has elapsed since the book was written, its mission, however, remains relevant today and the work continues to manifest its exemplary intellectual merit.

Marc Augé
Claudine Herzlich

INTRODUCTION

"The meaning of illness": the expression itself should be understood in at least two ways. Firstly, and this is true in any society, illness poses a problem, which requires interpretation. It must have a meaning if men are to have any hope of overcoming it. But this "meaning of illness", this interpretation developed within a society, can itself be studied and interpreted from a variety of viewpoints and that variety is duplicated in societies whose academic tradition has allotted its observation to different disciplines; to ethnology, for example, the observation of line-age-based societies; to sociology, that of industrial societies. The fact that these distinctions today are to a certain extent called into question is of little importance. They encourage a questioning of the relationships between the respective methods and objectives of the different disciplines. So the object before us here would be, so to speak, doubly duplicated. The local interpretation of illness is one thing, but it is quite possible that the interpretation of this interpretation could vary, depending on whether it was the product of different methods (anthropological, sociological, historical) or on whether it was applied to different societies. The situation may become even more complicated, since the question can always be raised as to whether types of method and types of society are mechanically linked, whether one type of society implies one type of method. Let us further confuse the issue by adding that ill, illness and ill-fortune are not a priori identical concepts. The very ambiguity of the term "ill", which can be taken in the physico-biological sense or in the moral and Christian sense, itself raises the historical problem of the transition from a perception of disease to an awareness of ill, a perception and an awareness which are far from being one and the same thing in those societies which have no great difficulty in establishing the disease-ill-fortune equation and simply treat illness from the intellectual point of view as one particular form of ill fortune.

A diversity of fields, a diversity of methods and viewpoints, a diversity in the concept: the meaning of illness seems to lose itself in the maze of disciplines, of cultures and of history. How are we to find our way out of the labyrinth?

In this book we have tried to take the shortest route. Many ethnologists whose major research interest was not illness or medicine have realized that they could not observe and try to understand the social, political or religious life of the communities that they were studying without taking account of their nosological systems as expressed in the manner of reaching diagnosis or therapeutic prescription, in the institutions which applied them or in the various agents involved in their application. In short, they could not do so without taking account of the social dimension of illness as expressed not only in the institutional structure and the ritual functioning of society but also in the intellectual models of the interpretation of reality of which this structure and this functioning are both the basis and one of the expressions. Certain historians, in particular those specializing in African studies, have been able to establish that endemic and, to a greater extent, epidemic illnesses (of which the prevention and treatment, if we are to believe ancient witness and ethnological observation, appear to be one of the main concerns of the religious and political leaders in the dynasties, the headships or the kingdoms) have both had an effect on and, conversely, have been affected by the social and political structuring of societies and their histories. Finally, it is also a fact that sociologists working in industrial societies have become aware in their various milieux of a certain number of similar phenomena, which can only be interpreted in relation to one another. It will be sufficient here to point out three of them. Illness acts as a social signifier; it is the subject of discourses which continually call into question the environment in the broadest sense of the word. These discourses vary according to the historical period and the social and professional situation of those who pronounce them. Finally, over the past twenty years we have seen a radically new phenomenon; the tendency of the discourse on health, both among those who have recourse to medicine and among the official representatives of medical policy, to talk in terms of health, rather than illness.

The social dimension of illness, then, was indeed the common characteristic of our different explorations. It remained for us to ask ourselves whether, from the intellectual and conceptual point of view, we were applying the terms "illness" and "social dimension" to uniform, or at least to comparable, realities. For years we have endeavoured to compare our experiences in the secret hope that, if the answer was in the affirmative, we would be able to benefit from our mutual contributions and, in particular, gain a better understanding of the efficiency of the interaction between the individual idealized image and social symbolism in the societies and cultures under observation. We hoped also to be able to contribute to the formulation of a transcultural theory on ideological efficacity. It is true that we have not yet achieved this, but we are justified in feeling that we have made some progress in establishing that we are indeed dealing with a conceptually coherent and uniform object in our attempts to define, as a result of our respective approaches, the "social dimension of illness".

Let us briefly outline the research and the results (albeit incomplete) that this book seeks to summarize, not by providing a compilation of more or less personal and disconnected data and reflections, but by reconstructing the progression, the logic and the spirit of a collective approach. The ethnologists, for their part, are here attempting to free themselves from the traditionally simplistic approach, which is based on the radical opposition between magical and rational thought and which gives pride of place to the diffusionist hypothesis in explaining the resemblances between cultures, (in this case between the nosological systems, aetiologies and therapeutic methods of different societies).

For Marc Augé, the anthropological viewpoint is not to be confused with the literal approach to the evolution of medical thought. The literal approach simply examines societies unequally placed on the axis of progress and depicts their rational accession to a knowledge of symptoms and aetiology. An over-dependence on this view precludes a thorough understanding of the social dimension of illness. The latter, perceived exclusively from an aetiological standpoint, becomes a relic of the "magical" mentality which is incapable of controlling disease by attributing it natural causes and by applying empirical treatment. This applies to all nosological systems, regardless of how "scientific" or efficient they are. More exactly, the latter, apprehended only in its aetiological aspect, is transformed into the vestige or the traces of a magical attitude of mind incapable of controlling illness by presupposing it to have natural causes and treating it empirically.

Now observation of the African situation (which American typologies tend to place in the magico-irrational category) shows at least that, on the one hand, illness in Africa is not social in the univocal sense of the word and that, on the other hand, consideration of its social dimension or dimensions excludes neither consideration of equilibriums between substances or between humours (which, as in Hippocrates' Greece, are supposed to guarantee health), nor recourse to plant remedies or therapeutic methods such as inoculation (which the evolutionist, topological and diffusionist approaches tend to consider as typical of a virtually empirico-rational sector and method). There is nothing, then, which fundamentally distinguishes the African systems from others and, on this point, Marc Augé disagrees with the analyses of an anthropologist like Foster who gives a distinct place to personalistic medical systems mainly on the grounds that they attribute all illness to the action of an external agent, be it man or god. What is interesting and important, however, is that even in African lineage-based societies, where the social aetiology of illnesses though not exclusive is certainly capital, illness is not social simply because of its presumed or sought cause. Using examples from the Ivory Coast or Togo, Marc Augé attempts to define this social character in relation to three "logics" and two "models". The logic "of differences" whose extent, rigour and complexity have been shown in several articles by Françoise Héritier, imposes an order based on equivalence or opposition, implication or exclusion, upon "the symbols which are used to think society and which constitute its intellectual structure." Cosmology, anthropology, meteorology, nosology or political theory do not belong to distinct intellectual categories and even if their common logic does not constitute a common unitary and truly closed discourse, it nevertheless furnishes the raw material and the implicit parameters of the juridical rules, cognitive principles and models of interaction peculiar to each society.

But ignoring the other two logics which dictate the definition, the interpretation and the history of illness would be to refrain from any sociological analysis of it. The logic of references dictates the distribution of the elements distinguished and ordered by the logic of differences in the realm of empirical social reality. It coincides to a large extent within a given society with the a priori set of interpretation norms which are usually grouped under the name of "social aetiology". However, everyone knows that the implementation of any theory, if it is to be effective (or at least harmless) to the one who formulates it, should take into account the strength of the (social) positions of the individuals concerned. The logic of references, of which the system of attitudes, dear to the ethnologist, or the general theories on witchcraft as they are occasionally referred to in monographs, give only a partial, general and dangerously uniform idea, (e.g. when we are told, for example, of the special respect that a son owes to his father in a matrilineal society and the possibility that the maternal uncle has in it to bewitch his uterine nephew) contains in fact all the multiplicity of positions of strength, of social situations and conditions in which authority may be exercised. Similarly, chronology, or logic of events, takes as axiomatic the need to consider simultaneously the evolution of the symptom itself and the reactions of the groups and the individuals that this evolution concerns.

The system, then, is never closed or rather, it can be indefinitely re-opened which is a consequence or an expression of what in Popper's language could be called its "non-falsifiable" character. A sign of this openness is the fact that there need not be total correspondence, for example, between diagnosis and therapy or between the analysis of the symptom and the establishing of the cause. In this connection, Marc Augé attempts to show how, in the voodoo systems of the Benin regions, there are two possible ways to arrive at a therapy, one of which gives first place to the symptom and the other to the cause. In the first it is the nature of the plants chosen to treat the symptom which, incidentally, entails the carrying out of rites and sacrifices to the gods who are their masters. In the second it is the identification by divination of the gods who are the causes of the illness, that provides the identification of the plants necessary for the cure irrespective of any symptomatological indication. The logic of differences which rules over the cosmological, theological or anthropological order, and which structures the symbolism of plants as well as that of the gods, the earth or the bodily humours is a principle of implicit coherence rather than an automatic source of reference to which should be related all the vicissitudes of individual or collective life.

Although illness is, in elemental form, an "event", in that its biological manifestations do not simply affect the body of an individual but are for the most part the object of social interpretation (bringing into play and often calling in question social relationships), it in no way follows that the ethnologist can analyse it in those societies where he works as he would a "medical system" in industrialised societies. Nicole Sindzingre insists on this point when she notes that identification and denomination of ailments, causality schemata and therapeutic institutions do not necessarily make a system. Even when it is possible to classify a certain number of facts into a series of causes or symptoms they cannot necessarily be confined in "hierarchic and inclusive taxonomies". Rather they are subject to the fluctuations of which Augé, as we have just seen, attempts to define the multiple possibilities and the retrospective necessities through the notions of "logic of parameters" and "chronologic".

Taking the Senufo as examples, Nicole Sindzingre analyses in depth the far from systematic nature of illness conceptions. This analysis gives pride of place to two perspectives ("the possible representations and practices of a priori causality" and "the exercise of a posteriori causality") and identifies three registers of coherence which dictate respectively the designation of ailments and their cause, their "miraculous" interpretation by divination, and the choice of the therapeutic procedures. This designation of the ailments and their cause comes within a priori causality which, itself, defines more an order of possibilities than a necessary order, as can be seen from both the instability of causal categories and the dissymmetry of the causality model and, more broadly, from the fluctuating relationship which specifically links the reading of the symptom to the determination of the cause. Causal categories are unstable. Responsible for providing an explanation not only for illness in particular but also for ill-fortune in general, they overflow freely into the field of religion and become identified with various figures or authorities which are associated with all the unknown dangers of social and religious life. God, twins or the dead in a matrilineage, the spirits of the bush or rivers, sorcerers, fetish objects, the *nyuma* of corpses are held to be responsible for certain types of illnesses, but a twin may be a form of ancestor or an ancestor may be a form of fetish. The causality model contains inherent contradictions: an event may be a posteriori related to one or another of the possible a priori causes (violation of a taboo or spell cast by a sorcerer, for example); on the other hand, the person who violates a taboo can expect to be the victim of ill-fortune and when this does occur it will have this cause, or another, assigned to it.

The relationship between symptom and cause fluctuates; although a certain number of symptoms may be associated with certain agents or certain forms of behaviour: coughing with God; stomach aches with violation of a taboo; leprosy with witchcraft. It is always possible to move from one cause to another when circumstances so require.

It is remarkable, however, that the two other registers of coherence (the effective interpretation of illness and therapy) do not necessarily depend on one another. The initial choice of one divinatory instrument or another indicates the type of causality likely to be preferred and the non-decisive role of the symptom at that moment testifies to the relatively lax character of the overall intellectual schema. Moreover, a form of divination like the *sandoho* which is widespread among the Senufo does not produce any form of therapy and, in general, Nicole Sindzingre can speak of the relative impermeability of the division between the interpretation register and the therapy register. Consequently, the development or the disruption of care techniques does not in itself entail a modification of the traditional explanatory models, "The (recognized) efficacity of Western biomedicine has no effect on causal thought since the primary function of the latter is not efficacity but explanation".

When she speaks of "invariants of symbolic thought", Françoise Héritier, whose main interest lies in representations of sterility, refers to three types of considerations. Firstly, even though the discourse on sterility is based on concrete observations, it speaks, above all, "of the social practice and the rules of behaviour relating to it". Secondly, since sterility is always and everywhere considered to be a feminine defect, it always tells us "something about the social relationships between the sexes". Finally, the discourse on sterility always postulates a homology "between the world, the individual body and society"; in fact, not only does it postulate this homology, it also implements it and functions to a certain degree as the operative element in the system of transformations which facilitates the movement from one register to another.

The truth is that the relationship between the natural universe, the individual body and society is not simply a homologous relationship. Each order has an effect on the other and the ultimate cause is always to be found in society, or at least in men whose errors or transgressions may produce an effect on individual bodies or on the world order. Let us take a few examples. Among the Samo of Upper Volta, the menses-less woman, the sterile woman *par excellence*, cannot be buried until her kidneys have been pierced through. This makes her blood flow and so prevents her corpse, which is bursting with hot blood, from drying up the earth (which by definition is hot) with an accumulation of heat when she is buried. Conversely, but this time within the register of relationships between successive generations, Françoise Héritier shows us the extreme ambiguity of relations between mother and daughter as expressed in the social rules which forbid them to be mothers at the same time, or at least forbid the mother to have a child so long as her daughter, once she is officially in a condition to do so, has not had her first child. Here again, sterility may be punishment for a transgression. All in all, and whatever the exceptions and the modalities, "crossing generations, crossing bloods, crossing genders" is a violation of the general order (simultaneously cosmic, individual and social), a violation whose immediate consequences, in particular drought and sterility, represent a spectacular warning (to those on whom they fall) to return to the pre-ordained order. The historian's contribution, here restricted to the African field, inclines the anthropologist to prudence and reflection. E. M'Bokolo, after having studied the nature and the interest of the various documents which may be of use in the writing of a history of certain epidemic and pandemic illnesses, goes on to a study of the two other fields in a possible history of illnesses. These are, firstly, the study of illnesses "in their relationship with economics and demography, which can be usefully based on existing works on historical demography, and medical geography, and, secondly, the study of illnesses in their multiple and complex relationships with global society". It is at this point and because of his need to study medical practices and knowledge that he comes to anthropological research. This affords the opportunity to give some useful warnings. For the difficulties which we see the historian encounter in his attempts to periodise the vast syntheses made by certain anthropologists are not merely the technical difficulties of a historian.

We all know that the notion of tradition, to the extent that it favours a uniform and a-historical conception of the past, is inadequate and dangerous. Illnesses, in particular, are sometimes datable and dated, they appear and they disappear, just like the changeable methods which are used to control or eliminate them. These methods, then, could not be the direct expression of an immutable wisdom and knowledge which is perennial and diffused throughout an entire society. But the historian, in absolving certain anthropologists from the sins of timelessness and uniformization, draws the attention of all of them to certain factual considerations.

E. M'Bokolo concentrates in particular on the example of the coastal regions of Africa which the historian can study in the light of the twofold contribution of travellers' tales and oral traditions. It is all the more remarkable then, that as far as they are concerned, the historian's approach, which is close to that of the anthropologist's, leads to markedly different conclusions. The differences would appear to concern three questions; the existence of specialists in medicine which the anthropologists tend to underestimate, the importance accorded in African societies to the preservation of health and to prevention (and not only to the interpretation of outbreaks of illnesses on which the anthropologists have concentrated), and finally, the collective organization of treatment and taking into care which the anthropologists appear to have rather overestimated.

On all these points it would seem that the historian's warnings are intended more to underline the need for a good anthropology than to stir up controversies between disciplines. As far as the last two points are concerned, we can bear in mind, (and Françoise Héritier's analysis helps us to do so) that there is no contradiction between the desire to ensure fertility (or to understand infertility and drought) and the desire to interpret illnesses, in particular since the idea that recovery of health in Africa traditionally requires the reconciliation of the individual with those close to him is derived from a subtly ethnocentric irenicism.

Nor is the existence of specialists questionable, even in non-statal societies, and the anthropologists do not dispute this. But E. M'Bokolo has in mind two types of analysis in particular which are indeed identified in anthropological literature. According to the first, African medical knowledge is, at the same time, spread throughout the whole social entity and preserved by a single specialized group, each expert intervening according to the nature, the seriousness or the course taken by the illness. According to the second type of analysis, medical knowledge does not delimit an independent intellectual area, but both by the nature of the ills to which it applies (ill-fortune in general) and by the nature of the causes which it reveals (which include the ill will of the gods or of men) it overflows into the realm of religion and politics. M'Bokolo does not deny that this is the case in certain places and at certain moments in history (in fact, he feels that the vulnerability of certain political powers to epidemics and to the subsequent swings of opinion is essential, as is the link between thaumaturgical power and political authority), but he casts doubt on the general nature of the schema and at the same time suggests that there is a genuinely medical tradition in Africa whose specificity is due at one and the same time to its objectives, its techniques and the agents which apply it. Neither Marc Augé nor Nicole Sindzingre would deny the first assertion which, in the formulation peculiar to the historian, seems to accord with one of their major concerns; namely, the need to denounce all closed generalisations and systematic conceptions of the ways illnesses and the methods of curing them are regarded in societies which cannot make an absolute distinction between the problems of meaning and the problems of knowledge (as in the case of industrial societies, for example).

The fact is that in Africa, as elsewhere, these problems can be considered from two distinct and complementary points of view. If we prefer the "meaning" viewpoint, we must admit (and this is the whole point of this book) that knowledge does not contain the whole of meaning and that, as far as we are concerned here, the impression of meaning produced by the interpretation of the illnesses and therapeutical practices does not depend on the supposed scientific nature of this interpretation. The anthropologists' first question, then, does not concern the truth or the efficacity of African medicine in such and such a place or at such and such a time, a question which most of them have no more the means to answer than their historian colleagues,[1] but, as we have said, it concerns its social dimension. The political and cultural variables highlighted in this respect by the historian undeniably enrich the definition of this dimension. If preference is given to the "knowledge" point of view, we will perhaps be more sensitive to the difference between two situations. It is current practice in Europe to contrast a more or less secret "popular" medicine with modern medicine. This type of contrast, possibly in more ecumenical forms, is becoming commonplace in Africa today. But prior to the introduction of Western medicine the contrast between the current conceptions of illness and those of the specialists was not of the same kind. Even when the knowledge was unevenly shared (a special place should doubtless be reserved for the examples of learned medicine found in certain royal courts which M'Bokolo mentions), they are not of a different nature, or rather, the difference between the layman and the specialist is more reminiscent of the difference which may exist between the average French executive with a vague idea of the properties of antibiotics and his doctor (or between a practising Catholic and his confessor) than of the difference between the modern doctor and the healer in a Norman or Lorraine village. Agreeing on the general meaning of knowledge, the layman and the specialist only differ in the inequality of their knowledge. So it is the exact nature of this blend of meaning and knowledge characteristic of the non-specialist's conceptions which poses the problem. In our opinion, however, this problem concerns the users of the health institution in 20th century Paris as much as it does the users of Ashanti medicine in the 18th or 19th centuries. It is also different from the problem presented in both Africa and Europe (under different conditions it is true), by the coexistence of several medical traditions, which, in the light of modern medicine's tendency toward monopoly as far as knowledge is concerned, doubtlessly induces the "different" medicines to lay claim to the exclusivity of meaning.

All in all, in this collection, the harmony between anthropologists and historians is deep-rooted. They all know that illness, like death, is a good subject for reflection, and that many political leaders know this from bitter experience. The tension between disciplines, in principle salutary, is due to the fact that the anthropologist gives preference to the analyzable effects of meaning in the societies which he is studying (though he is sometimes tempted, it must be admitted, into a somewhat undisciplined comparativism), whereas the historian distinguishes behind the ideological facade, the materials of the various ages which have constructed it and seeks the meaning of the whole in the successive reasons for this construction. That each society and each period of history have different characteristics and that consequently each one of them may be the place or the occasion for a more or less baroque accumulation of original elements and diverse purposes is something that anthropology sometimes, though unwittingly, gives the impression of concealing because it is first and foremost interested (as it thinks are those who live there), in the overall aspect (we do not say the homogeneity) of the societies which it studies. It does indeed need the historian to remind it, if it is not to lose sight of its objective, that just like individuals and societies, representations, concepts, systems and gods belong to an age.

The same warning is valid for sociology. Although it succumbs less than anthropology to the temptation of the overall view, and it has learned to a certain extent to take account of history in the analysis of present day industrial society, it does neglect the history of other kinds of society. It can even be said that, at least for quite some time, the comparison of industrial society with others was reduced in one way or another to a contrast between what changes, what evolves or advances, and what remains or stagnates. For a long time sociologists held that the others had no history. This is where E. M'Bokolo's analysis obliges the sociologist of medicine and illness to radically call things into question. For the sociologist concerned, whatever his distance from the triumphalism of a certain medical philosophy, the 19th century was a period of undeniable progress in knowledge and of increasing efficacity in medical and health intervention. During this period the major epidemics in Europe were finally overcome. In Africa, however, M'Bokolo shows us that the period of the greatest colonial penetration, which was also the period of the penetration of Western medicine, was "the time of death", the time of the spreading of epidemics and of demographic collapse. We can see graphically the disastrous nature of certain of the interventions engendered by Western medical logic and scientific theory when they are introduced outside the society which produced them. We can appreciate then, not only that the history of others does exist but also that it can be different from ours – and this is true of the colonial period in Africa.

For the sociologist working on industrial societies, the study of lineage-based societies is fascinating. First of all because of its overabundance of meanings, its multiplicity and wealth of interpretations, the variety of which seems to warn us against the danger of becoming confined in the rigidity of a closed system. It is necessary, however, to advance beyond these first, perhaps ingenuous fascinations and attempt to discover more fundamental similarities and divergences. It is also necessary to clearly identify the hypotheses which, though based on different grounds, materials and problematics may allow a convergent construction. We began, in fact, with two working hypotheses; in the first place that there is no need to postulate the absolute heterogeneity of industrial and lineage-based societies: secondly, that in spite of its importance, modern medicine does not introduce into thinking about illness a division of such an extent that it becomes devoid of any social dimension. The viewpoint of truth is not extra-social. Rather is it the sociologist's ambition to construct an analysis where "medicine", its knowledge and its praxis, is itself integrated into the social dimension of illness.

Claudine Herzlich analyses how this problem has been approached hitherto by sociology and she makes a distinction between two trends of research. The first was marked by the sociologist's acceptance of the medical definition of illness, a biological fact affecting the individual's body and decoded by medicine. The social dimension of illness, then, is but the series of factors which affect the initial biological fact but without transforming its nature. For other writers, however, the relationship between organic state and socially recognized illness is not one of simple continuity; "health" and "illness" are in themselves social categories which have been constructed by medical knowledge and practice. The sociologist's task, then, is to understand the mechanisms, the role and the effects of this construction.

Both of these approaches, however, have neglected one problem. It is true that in industrial societies illness is essentially a matter for the doctor and for medicine. But it is never that alone. It is not just a series of symptoms which makes us go and see the doctor. It still remains an unhappy event requiring an interpretation which is never simply individual. The interpretation is collective, shared by members of the same social group, but it is also an interpretation which, in the strict sense of the expression, calls society into question and says something of our relationship with society. The social dimension of illness, — and this is where sociology joins anthropology — lies in the fact that it functions as a signifier, the basis of the meaning of our relationship with society.

The empirical analysis of conceptions of illness and health in our society provides confirmation of this point of view. Using a study carried out during the 1960s among members of the middle classes, executives and professionals, Claudine Herzlich shows how these conceptions are expressed in a language which is not that of the body but of the relationship between the individual and society. From the aetiological angle in particular, illness is ascribed to society's aggressiveness, which imposes an unhealthy "life-style" on the individual. Illness, from the objective, and hence corporeal, viewpoint, incarnates our conflictive relationship with society. In a recent study on conceptions of health, Janine Pierret finds themes of the same nature. These conceptions reveal to us a coherence in social and symbolic practices ordered by reference to the signifier, health. Through it the members of the various social groups express their relationship, not only with work and consumption, but also with time, social space and nature.

A first conception is centred on the deterioration of the body-illness – and is linked to a set of themes concerning excesses and abuses, mainly in eating habits, as opposed to balance and moderation. Another, widespread among the working classes, considers health to be a fundamental asset, built up in childhood and related to the obligation to engage in work and activity. It can be noted that this conception of health is close to certain African conceptions of fertility described by Françoise Héritier (but in the lineage-based societies this store of vital force belongs to the generation and not to the individual). But health can also be seen as the yardstick which dictates the organization of all individual practices, in particular consumption habits, in a constant dialectic between what is, for the individual, controllable or uncontrolled, between the private and the public, between pleasure and risk. Finally, for others, who are usually young, graduates and middle or senior cadres, the notion of health is seen primarily as an object for State responsibility and intervention.

These conceptions allow us to identify the elements of a sort of common code which is the basis (with differing arrangements in the various social groups but according to regulated variations) for all our reasoning and daily practices related to health and illness. In conjunction with this research, the works of anthropologists on lineage-based societies help us achieve a better understanding of the nature of our collective reasoning, of our social thinking on illness. They then lead us to reconsider the role of medicine, its institution and its knowledge, in the way the West conceptualizes and assumes responsibility for illness, health and bodily phenomena. Let us first of all note, at the most general level, the similarity between "modern" reasoning and that of societies that are still sometimes called "primitive". When they talk about illness and health, sociologists can perfectly well adopt for themselves, for example, what Françoise Héritier says about sterility; "these conceptions are not based on scientific knowledge, they emanate from social practice and the rules of behaviour relating to it".

Moreover, the conceptions which we have mentioned may also be ordered according to Marc Augé's classification of a logic of differences, references and events. For us, too, illness is apprehended as an event. Furthermore, the "unhealthy life style" as opposed to the "healthy life", "natural" as opposed to "chemical" food constitute dichotomies comparable to the symbolic categories (dry and wet, hot and cold, whose importance is shown by Françoise Héritier) of the African logic of differences. The order of references, that of the balance of power or social relationships is also at the heart of our conception of illness. As we have said, it is a state of society and of our relationship to it that is expressed by our vision of the biological. At this level, then, there is no heterogeneity between the modes of thought of the two types of society.

Similarly, we can easily find in our conceptions examples of that circular thought analysed by Nicole Sindzingre who shows that the society she is studying is less interested in establishing schemata of causality than in emphasizing a world order in which the individual has his place. The same element, can be used either a priori with a causal and predictive value for a specific event or a posteriori as the reconstituent interpretation of the past. In the conceptions of illness, of health, or of cure analysed by Claudine Herzlich, Janine Pierret and Danièle Léger, the notion of "life style" or of "modern society" is a principle of coherence which can, in the same way, function circularly when the aim is to establish the various relationships between the biological and the social. Regarded as the specific cause of certain ailments, the modern life style is also at the basis of the a posteriori global reinterpretation of any failure of the body. Here again the question is less of providing an accurate list of causes than of decoding meaning. As the expression of our unsatisfactory relationship with society, the "modern lifestyle" cannot be invalidated.

It is possible, however, to find a marked difference between the two modes of thought. In the conceptions of lineage-based societies the logic of differences and the logic of references appear interwoven in the same system of symbolic opposition. As Marc Augé states explicitly, "the social references, as we have seen, bring into play a symbolism of the same kind as that which dictates the "natural" relationships between hot and cold, dry and wet, etc." Françoise Héritier's analysis shows this particularly well, "fertility and sterility transcribe the relationships between generations as far as the body is concerned. The world, the individual body and society are homologous in nature". The logic of differences which operates in our conceptions constitutes rather a series of oppositions applicable to the natural order but where the social relationships are, in fact, in concrete form, naturalized. In this sense the logic of differences does indeed show us society but in a transformed form, as the material conditions surrounding us. The "social" aspect has to become material and so become part of nature, even if it is to corrupt it. It must become objectivized in "chemical" food and pollution if the body is to be affected by it. Where the symbolic order of the lineage-based society seems to unify two orders of reality, ours translates, establishes correspondences, interaction and transformations. This passage from one register to another demands, moreover, a key, namely the abstract notion of "society" which is omnipresent in all our conceptions, and which is essential in objectivizing the social dimension. Bearing in mind this observation, we will perhaps become more aware of the strength of the division that we are establishing when we think in terms of social and natural relationships.

We then gain a better understanding of the role played by the development of specialized medical knowledge, situating the decoding of illness at the organic level alone. On the one hand it has cut the link between the description of the organic illness and the order of references, the organic is divorced from the social. It has, moreover, developed a system of categories which the logic of differences, the body of symbols which has become a system of concepts, is supposed to be more than a simple reading, an objective decoding of the event. It is perhaps these divisions and these limitations which make interpretation difficult for us; there is little free room for working on meaning. This seems to be the price that we have to pay for the knowledge that we have acquired.

Nicole Sindzingre's analysis of the dissociation between the interpretation of illness and its therapy among the Senufo reveals another aspect. In Europe, today, these two levels always operate in close association. The whole development of Western medical thought is embodied in the endeavour to attain this coincidence between the interpretation of symptoms, the discovery of a causality and the implementation of a therapy. The Pasteurian notion of specific aetiology, where the link is as close as possible between the symptom, the microbial agent and the action on this agent marks one of the most outstanding periods of this development. Modern medicine has inculcated in us this integration which, today, can be found in the "lay" conceptions which we have analysed. Biological illness is the signifier of our unsatisfactory relationship with society, through it we express a weariness with life or a values crisis, but our conception of it first of all takes the form of a causal theory; modern life style engenders illnesses. Here meaning is hidden under cause, or rather it can only find expression in seeking a cause.

Yet we know that today medicine itself is dissatisfied with the closed nature of its conceptual system, modern theories of illness in particular have abandoned all simple causal models.[2] They are multi-linear, admitting a series of different factors in a complex interaction. As for lay thought, the conception of illness as a social ill goes far beyond any attempt at making an exhaustive list of causalities. When we speak of illness as being produced by society we do not just intend to add to its aetiological model social or psychological factors which might be forgotten by the organicist approach. Through this identification of a causal factor we are giving much wider expression to the crisis of meaning in present day society. Health, illness, the body are treated in it as metaphoric objects, the bases and crystallization of the most acute questioning of social evolution.

This is particularly clear in the study of groups and practices (such as those of the apocalyptic neo-rural communities analysed in this work by Danièle Léger) in which illness and health constitute one of the stages necessary for the most extreme form of questioning of the social order. In these small neo-rural communities, after a return to "nature", to a "healthy" and "natural" life based on ecological conceptions, there is a gradual build-up of the vision of an imminent planetary disaster which would wipe out our industrial society based on artificiality and the destruction of nature. The corollary to this collective apocalypse is illness, its equivalent at the individual level, the revenge-punishment of a nature which man had wrongly thought that he could ill-treat indefinitely. It is also a sign and a call to order; man today is suffering from the modern world which he has created but illness tells him that this world will be destroyed tomorrow.

So in this case a system of beliefs and notions, which we recognize are linked to a common conception, is at the root of breakdowns and radical questioning. These groups are preparing for the apocalypse and are trying to organize conditions for survival. These communities' search for "natural" behaviour, their rejection of modern medicine is at the same time an attempt to cure the body, to reconstruct the meaning of individual and collective behaviour and to establish a group survival strategy. Just as illness and medicine metaphorize the artificial and condemned modern world so the notion of curing metaphorizes both that of survival and of salvation.

One may be tempted to draw a parallel between these communities and the case of certain groups of sick people analysed by Claudine Herzlich. These groups, which have been growing for several years, are trying to find "other ways" of healing than those of modern medicine. They often start from a neo-hippocratic conception of the "force of nature", of the "resistance" of the individual as an essential weapon against illness which comes from the aggression of society. But groups of sick people and apocalyptic communities are, in a certain sense, taking an opposite direction. For the communities, the disaster which is threatening the world is also expressed at bodily level. For sick people, it is the sometimes imminent disaster that attacks the organism which comes first: the quest for meaning has the body's weakness and not the disorder in the world as its starting point. But it also implies a questioning of the social dimension. The medicine which these sick people refuse because they feel it is ineffective and even harmful, is the particularly alienating and dangerous expression of a harmful society. The sick, then, struggle against their illness, against medicine and against a society which legitimizes medicine and expresses itself through it.

If we return for an instant to the communities studied by Danièle Léger we can easily observe that with them and in them comes to an end the circular path which has led us from the lineage-based societies and the kingdoms of Africa to the vicissitudes of industrial society. In these communities which grow up around a salvation ideal to escape the deleterious vices of the civilisation of towns and factories, illness still has to be understood when it appears, re-calling its existence to those who had thought that they were sheltered from it and who interpreted their new immunity as a sign or a promise of salvation. In this case, illness can only have the effect of a call to order: "illness in such a context can no longer be considered, as it usually is in the dominant society, as an insane and intolerable accident: it may be collectively and individually experienced as an indicator of unresolved tensions within the group or within the relations of the group with its territory". Once again the group is constantly made known to itself through the intermediary of the bodies of those who constitute it: the inscription of (social) meaning on the (individual) body is immediate.

But, if the viewpoints of the anthropologist and the sociologist readily converge on this paradoxical response of the lineage-based or village societies, to the point where they seem to be almost identical, they usually discover, in their respective objectives, not areas of identity, it is true, but areas of comparison, intellectual landscapes which recall each other even in their differences. For to suggest, as we have just done, that the ethnological analyses offer to the sociologist points of view and notions which he can adopt even if they have to be adapted to his own devices, is also to admit that, conversely, the matter and the method of the sociologist may usefully inspire the anthropological project.

To put it in a nutshell, we can say that what is explicit in one discipline corresponds to what is implicit in the other. Elements which are implicit, but decodable in the industrial society (Claudine Herzlich shows us this) are the representations of illness as deviance, the demand for meaning which overflows or informs knowledge, the definition of the role of sick people as a social role: the explicit element is the conception of their illness by individuals whose oral expression of it is often the starting point for sociological analysis. This is how the anthropologist, as in a mirror placed behind his usual object of observation, sees the image of its hidden face. For the intimate expression of his feelings by the sick subject is precisely what the anthropologist of different cultures finds most difficult to accede to, for several reasons, in particular those which result from differences between languages, the difficulties of silence and allusion, the difficulty also of establishing a personal relationship with a sufficient number of individuals to make communication possible, comprehensible and significant. On the other hand, in the societies in which the social anthropologist works, the main lines of the system by which illnesses are interpreted are usually official and sufficiently well known to be the subject of a general conception as are political or religious organizations. So the sociologist can take as his objective (as does Janine Pierret in this book) the revelation of the implicit system which can be distinguished, more or less clearly, in the discourse of the inhabitants of a housing estate in the Essonne and the farm workers in the Herault, although it may mean becoming interested in the constituents and the determinants of the system(s), whereas the social anthropologist starts from the system to attempt to grasp its meaning and show its effects, in particular on the behaviour and speech of individuals, even if doing so means casting doubt on the truly systematic character of the system.

Often the social anthropologist only observes those elements of the system referred to as are revealed by an account which shapes and transforms it (if it does not actually annihilate it). Hence he is tempted to "reconstitute" it and, in so doing, if he does not pay attention to the warnings of the historian, to freeze it in an artificial, idealised synchronism. But here again the analysis proposed by the sociologists of a reality closer in time (and closer to him since it is his own) can help him to take into consideration the speed with which illness can change its meaning. Claudine Herzlich shows how in certain groups and particularly in society as a whole, which every day is becoming increasingly cost-conscious, health is increasingly presented to the sick individual as "his business", which implies that any illness that he may suffer will also be his business, his bad luck and, ultimately, his fault. This new highlighting of an incessant tension between meaning and knowledge should encourage the social anthropologist not to succumb to the temptation to reduce this tension to a simple conflict between traditional knowledge and modern knowledge, unequally perceived and recognized.

All in all, then, the aim of this book is to help to reveal the relationship between anthropological, historical and sociological "disciplines" when they are applied to the same task. This relationship is neither exclusive nor truly complementary. The disciplines differ in their methods, of course, but also in the objectives which they set themselves and which, in a sense, they construct. The respective goals of anthropology, history and sociology do not blend into one another but they partially overlap and the social dimension of illness seems to us to be an area of overlap which each discipline envisages from its own point of view. To be aware of this diversity is, for each of them, to be more acutely aware of its particularity. They all have to avoid the temptation of disciplinary and falsely theoretical monolithism. There is no contradiction in being interested in both the constants of symbolic thought and in the fact that systems and societies change, nor is it aberrant to analyse the specific rationality of the effects of meaning without ignoring, for all that, the relationship between those forces which constitute social history or (to return more exactly to the subject which interests us here), the impressive progress of modern medical knowledge.

NOTES

1. Though ethnomedical research of the past few years could be enlightening in this respect in so far as it is not satisfied with drawing up lists of plants even when they are identified.
2. We could refer, for example, to present debate between geneticists and psychoanalysts on the causes of mental illness. Cf. Claire Brisset "Psychoanalyse génétique." *Le Monde*, 16 December 1981, p 21.

Part I

BODILY AILMENTS, LINEAGE LANGUAGE

Chapter 1

BIOLOGICAL ORDER, SOCIAL ORDER: ILLNESS, AN ELEMENTAL FORM OF EVENT

M. AUGÉ

One would like, under this too ambitious title, to examine a theoretical hypothesis and the African experience which occasioned it.

The occasion first of all: it is the observation made during investigations in the lagoon zone of the Ivory Coast, then in the south of Togo, about the important role played by the interpretation of illness and misfortune in the life of lineal societies, the social questions (perhaps one should write the *question of society*) which follow manifestations of biological disorder. The systems of interpretation, possibly used by specialists but known or at least recognised by everybody, in fact make any biological disorder the sign of social disorder, such as aggression in witchcraft, adultery, the breaking of a taboo, etc. In the world of the lagoon, these questions can very naturally cause confrontations between groups or within groups. These confrontations play a substantial part in village or inter-village social activity and they contribute in a certain way to the definition of social units or sub-units which they oppose and which ethnology recognizes when it speaks of difficult relations between a maternal uncle and uterine nephew in a matrilineal system or the tension between allied lineages in all systems as a structural effect.

The hypothesis is that the same intellectual logic controls the biological order and the social order; that in some way, in a given society, a single interpretive framework of the world applies as much to the individual body as to social institutions. If there is a logic, it is from this very thing that the constitution of the body and the institution of society, the one and the others, simultaneously proceed.

1. ILLNESS AS AN ELEMENTAL FORM

It is the very paradox of illness that it is at one and the same time the most individual and the most social of things. Each one of us feels it in his body and sometimes dies from it. By feeling illness threatening and growing within him, an individual can feel cut off from others, from everything which makes his social life. At the same time everything about illness is social, not just because a certain number of institutions take it in charge at the different phases of its evolution, but because the patterns of thought which allow one to recognize it, to identify and treat it are eminently social: to think about one's illness is already to make reference to others.

This aspect is particularly obvious in African lineal societies where illness often has the value and meaning of a social call to order which itself entails a redefinition of the individual. It can signal an attack, a set-back, an error or a choice, but in each case comes back to a coded deciphering of symptoms which brings into question one or several pertinent social dimensions. The attack can, according to the society, emanate from inside or outside the lineage, but it can never be the deed of just any individual and consequently is only understood in relation to political and social organisation. The idea that the patient himself may have tried to attack another but failed, is also well attested and goes back to definitions of the person, of psychic entities, of the forces which attach to them, which are at the same time social definitions because they entail ideas of heredity, age, circumstances of birth, etc. Illness due to a personal mistake (lack of respect for an elder, neglect of a taboo) or to a mistake of others (receipt of a name which fails to take into account the partial reincarnation of an ancestor, being deceived by one's wife) is obviously socially coded. It is even more so when it has to be interpreted as the call of a God to serve him.

So the example of illness demonstrates in a remarkable way that there is no merely individual thought (let us at once understand about and by a single individual). In African or Amerindian creation myths, the birth of humanity is at the same time the birth of society. There is here an irreducible fact which sufficiently expresses (or is sufficiently expressed by) the necessary alienation from the institution from which Castoriadis[1] makes a law of *social imagination* and which seems the condition of all thought. Here we touch upon the problem of symbolic or ideological efficiency.

This problem itself can be formulated in at least two ways, culturally and also with a more universal end. Firstly one can ask oneself why the sum of determinants of a cultural configuration does not account for all the aspects of this configuration. It is thus that Castoriadis asks himself at the same time why it is in imagination that a society has to seek "the complement necessary for its order" and why there is always found "at the heart of this imagination and through all its expressions, something which cannot be reduced to functionality which is like an initial investment of the world and of oneself through society with a meaning which is not dictated by real factors since it is rather it which confers such importance and such a place in the universe which this society constitutes onto these real factors" — a sense quite close, as Castoriadis points out, to what Hegel called "the spirit of a people" (p. 179). Social imagination thus culturally marked is distinguished from the functional, as culture from ideology in the analysis which Establet[2] proposes a little after Castoriadis. Quite remarkably in fact, and although it was inspired more clearly and more explicitly by Althusserian Marxism, this analysis also finishes by making evident behavioural norms which are not directly socially determined. Establet criticises the notion of culture as understood by American culturalism in its entirety and notably Herskovitz ("the sum of behavioural models present in a defined society") because of a lack of specificity in his field of action ("... the cultural, like the behavioural models of which it is the sum, is distributed over all instances of social formation.... From the material base to ideology, all social structures pass through it"). On the contrary, Establet attempts to identify an autonomous cultural dimension which would rather belong to the realm of values. In fact he opposes culture in the strict sense, understood as that part of behavioural norms not directly determined socially (how, in another hypothesis, could the phenomena of ostentatious consumption be understood? he asks himself), and society as "the sum of objective structures which distribute the means of production and power between individuals and social groups and which determine social, economic and political practices". A pattern is thus elaborated which essentially respects the verticality of instances (where the social determined by the economic controls practice and forms ideology) while taking its somewhat marginal place on a side-branch of the superstructure within culture, the wild flower of ideology whose colours can vary from one social formation to another. Perhaps one can perceive in this language the recognition of a limit and the acknowledgement of a malaise. The recognition of a "surplus", of a "remainder" which escapes socio-economic determinism and cannot be pigeon-holed the framework of instances doubtless marks the limits of a metaphor and warns against mechanistic utilisation.

But one can also ask, or rather one is obliged to ask (and it is the essential merit of Castoriadis' most fertile intuitions) what is the motivating force behind alienation from institutions, without stopping at the simple fact that this alienation can take particular forms in different societies. Recognizing, like Lévi-Strauss, that an economic organisation, a legal system, an institutional power, a religion "exist socially as sanctioned symbolic systems", but in also describing the symbolic as at the same time composed imaginatively and subject to the imagination, "the root of alienation as well as creation in history" (p. 186), Castoriadis introduces two essential questions, one about the reason why the oppressed remain bound to a myth which they fight against or denounce (and which corresponds to a fundamental arbitrariness, in the sense of any institutionalised social form), the other on why the dominant groups are relatively alienated from the institutions upon which their domination is founded. The answer to these two questions is not really given (assuming it could be) and these are even imperceptibly changed when one contends oneself with evoking the irreducible, not to say incomparable and untranslatable, nature of the mythic forms in each particular, concrete culture.

Here we propose to embark on a modestly empirical way of proceeding, examining realities which might offer a concrete content for analysis of the notion of effectiveness. It seems to us the sum of these realities coming from what one could call "elemental forms of event", understanding by this term all the individual, biological events whose interpretation, imposed by the cultural model, is immediately social. Birth, illness, death are, in this sense, "elemental" events.

These elemental forms are simultaneously individual and social forms *par excellence*, which lend themselves at the same time to a particular, symbolic treatment. The parallel with symbolised forms of event (initiation, enthronement) seems not only possible, but obvious, and it is often said of these institutions that they are the occasion for the individual of the death of a former existence or a rebirth to his new life, and for societies the occasion of a return to its origins and of a rejuvenation. Ultimately, the relation between elemental forms and symbolic forms seems to be able to be read equally in either sense, like a reciprocal, metaphoric relation: birth and death are in some way initiation trials, the occasion of rites of passage from one state to another. Elemental events and symbolised events moreover have a fundamental and essentially paradoxical, common characteristic: unique to the individual (one only lives once, as one only dies once), they are essentially recurrent (and beyond that ritual) for all others; the diary is the same day to day. Elemental events simply correspond to the crux of this paradox: the individual did not see himself being born, he is not present at his burial but it is precisely at the moment when he emerges from nothing or he disappears back, that he is the object of the most intense socialisation, the one which marks crucial points in the collective life of the living adults.

Illness is the individual and social reality closest to these two essential moments. Moreover it can catapult them against each other by a short circuit effect which societies with a high infant mortality know well. Illness is regression, threat of death. But he who comes through it, as one says, feels reborn. It is trial *par excellence* and, generally, the occasion of great social activity. So it is not surprising that all societies have elaborated on it more or less sophisticated pronouncements. These pronouncements have at least three common features:

1) They speak about the individual (his definition, his make-up, his fate and what has befallen him);

2) They speak of society (the social causes of illness, threats to social values and situations structurally determined in terms of heredity, kinship, alliance, etc.);

3) They are partly based on factual observation: symptoms and circumstances of the illness.

The analysis of illness, as an elemental form, ought to take into account the triple constraint which controls interpretation. This triple constraint is a matter on one side of the circumstances of the event and the autonomy of sequences of events in relation to interpretations which attempt to understand and control them, on the other side of the internal cohesion of symbolic and intellectual patterns which serve as interpretations, finally of the existence of an already thought out social order, symbolised and institutionalised prior to the event, which constitutes in relations of force the relations of meaning described by these patterns.

The necessarily social content of any definition of illness is perhaps

easier to understand in medical (and social) systems which posit more
explicitly than others the existence of a link of a natural kind between
nosology and the social order. Luc de Heusch,[3] enquiring into the
reasons why man has been able to try to think of his individual fate
within the categories of his social surroundings, the reasons why "nosology" and "religion" are linked in numerous societies, has evoked "the
painful contradiction between the relative permanence of social being
and the irremediable fragility of individual being". One could add,
depending on the facts, that the terms of the link are not simply nosology
and religion, the latter obviously not being independent, neither in its
intellectual organisation nor in its functioning, from the rest of society,
and, depending on the cause, that it is not possible for historic, concrete
man to think of his "individual fate" in ways other than he does already;
moreover it cannot be taken as read that thought of his fate is foremost
in man; it occasions speculation and systems only in a secondary manner
with particular individuals. The ritual machinery of religion seems more
called upon to understand and direct events than to construct a medita-
tion on the meaning of life and this could appear, indirectly, in the eyes
of the observer who is studying the constants and themes of the ritual
system. For all that it is not the latter's primary goal. As for the "relative
permanence of social being", it defines itself through social institutions
which are also intellectual constructions implying an often differential
definition of the person (lineage, heritage, name alliance, succession, age
status, etc.). Social being would not have a relative permanence if its
definition did not imply a certain relativity and, as a corollary, a relative
permanence of the individual (relativity and permanence which are
expressed in universally spread theories of the individual as a composite
sum of elements or principles, possibly transmissible or inheritable).
Such and such an individual could well "build this up" and find conso-
lation in the idea that he will survive in the person of his children or
through the transmission of his patrimony, but this feeling, which cannot
explain the character of institution whose existence he presupposes, is
only the individual, affective translation of intellectual patterns which
individual and social thought inscribe in the same logical continuity.
This continuity, once again, is perhaps more easily perceptible in societies where the social dimension of nosology is more explicit, but there is
no society where it does not allow itself to be understood, thus display-
ing the vital, sociological minimum common to any society which wishes
that any thought on the individual, is also a thought on society.

   Now the existing literature hardly helps the exploration of this proposition. Sometimes in effect, principally in medical histories, it presents

social rootedness as the primitive, magical strait-jacket from which empirical medicinal would be progressively released; sometimes, under the label "medical anthropology" or "ethnomedicine" it shows us how indigenous taxonomies correspond more to a classification of supposedly social causes than a systematic ordering of symptoms, finally sometimes, under the same label, it completes this presentation by work which tries to measure the degree of objective effectiveness of local therapeutics, to identify the plants used, to recognize the physical area of certain illnesses and to record the types of indigenous diagnostics and treatments.

The results of some of this research are incontestable, but one could ask oneself if they are, properly speaking, anthropological. In measuring the interest of local systems from the point of view of scientific truth and, to some extent, from the point of view of medicinal rather than from the point of view of illness, one almost necessarily promotes an evolutionist perspective and a critical regard which considers the attempts of others as so many unequal efforts to approach Western type effectiveness. That said, it is not a matter here of denouncing Western centricity in the name of a cultural relativism which in any event is inappropriate, but to remember that the point of view of scientific truth, in these matters, obliges one to treat as a survival or an insufficiency proper to a certain state of society, which is precisely what creates the sociological interest in the phenomenon of illness, to know its social character, in all senses. Not that this last point cannot vary with the society where one observes it (doubtless, for example, one could make a distinction, under this aspect, between civilisations which begin by teaching men to silence their bodies in order to control them and those which teach them to listen to them to survive); but this social character, under its different modalities, remains the fundamental paradox of illness in all societies. If one wished to call it "magic", it must then be said that the task of the anthropology of illness is less about distinguishing, within primitive societies, between magic and empiricism, than about recognizing, in any society and independently of the degree of objective effectiveness of its medicinal, the "magical" (social) part in any illness.

The "point of view of truth", however, recognizes, even if it considers it as an ephemeral, twilight zone, the social dimension of illness. By the same token it allows one to clarify the difficulties which attach to its analysis. It is thus that an historian like Sigerist in *A History of Medicine*,[4] to account for an evolution which does not begin with nothingness, bases his analysis of ancient medicine on two distinctions (between causes and symptoms on one hand and magic and empiricism on the others, which the most recent anthropology seems to go on rediscovering without being able to go beyond them.

In Ancient Egypt, when magical, religious and empirical, rational elements were closely associated, one distinguishes three types of healer: the doctor, the Sekhmet priest and the sorcerer. If the distinction between magical, religious medicinal and empirical, rational medicinal to a large extent is covered by the one established quite naturally between etiology and symptomatology, it is because magical, religious therapy is first of all etiological, operating by expelling the demon or the ancestor which it considers the cause of the pain, whereas in empirical, rational therapy the illness is identified with the symptom which material remedies, such as plants, can make disappear. As for the distinction between magic and religion, it is seen by Sigerist, following Rivers, under its technical aspect, sorcerers introducing an object into the body of their victim or taking away one of his "souls" when spirits penetrate the body or attack him from outside. For certain professional anthropologists of the Christian religion, the distinction between magic and religion marks the point of cleavage between good and bad tendencies in primitive thought, at one and the same time because religion is on the side of the social structure that it expresses and magic alongside this structure, nonetheless vulnerable to its action, and because religion carries a portion of truth (measured against Christianity) of which magic is the perversion (and fetishism the expression). Such is one of the important conclusions of Father Tempels at the end of his analysis of Bantu thought.[5] For medical science, also evolutionist in this sense, the cleavage would seem somewhat higher, between magical, religious techniques in their entirety and empirical, rational symptomatology, nevertheless mixed in Egyptian practice, like the good grain and the chaff.

In this mixture social connections are uncovered and deciphered as a survival (or a sin) whereas they are part of the definition of illness in general (and therefore also of medicinal) just as its irreducible portion of political effectiveness and sociological meaning. The historical perspective of medicinal, because it is situated on the technical level, does not inform us about the conceptual and symbolic modalities through which the social informs the grasp of the biological.

Historical evolutionism has anthropological typologisms its counterpart. We will take for example an article by George M. Foster[6] which proposes a theoretical synthesis of great scope and a new way of research to escape from the painstaking but reduced and often repetitive descriptions of medical ethnography. Foster starts with the idea that the etiology of illness provides the key to comparisons between non-Western medical systems. The consideration of cultural diversity allows him, he thinks, to contest the claim according to which religion and medicinal would always be intimately linked: this link for him is only one cultural possibility among others. On the other hand, what the literature on the subject shows is that the modes of diagnostic and techniques of care and prevention are linked to the social configuration as a whole, this link itself being a function of the beliefs bearing on the causes of illness.

Under this relation, Foster distinguishes two main types of medical system, according to which they are "personalistic" or "naturalistic". In the first, the illness would be attributed to the active and deliberate intervention of a human, non-human (ancestor, spirit) or supernatural (God) agent, whose victim the patient would be. The illness would only appear as one feature of misfortune. The medical and religious practices would be tightly knit together at the same time. The causes of the pain would be understood at several levels, as Evans-Pritchard has well demonstrated concerning the Azande. The therapy ought to be active and positive to ward off the aggressor or expel the pain. The responsibility for the pain would be out of the victim's control. In systems of the second type, on the other hand, the illness would generally be attributed to the influence of natural forces of elements, such as cold, warmth, damp, dryness, etc., and more precisely to a loss of the balance which controls the reciprocal relations of the body's constituents. The balance of humours or principles of the yin and yang type would moreover be a function of the age and condition of the individual. The illness would have nothing to do with the other categories of misfortune; magic and religion would play no role in the therapeutic. The causes of the pain would not be ascribable on several levels. Illness would be avoided more than cured and the cure would not be achieved through the struggle with an aggressor. The responsibility of the patient would always be involved when an illness broke out. The whole of this nosologic and medical tradition would be common to Greece, Rome, India and China, whereas the "personalistic" pattern would be evidenced in Africa. One finds the same kind of inspiration in the Murdock[7] school which is based on a sample of 139 societies belonging to 6 large, different, cultural regions. Murdock, after having distinguished the theory of natural causality (and its 5 types) and the theory of supernatural causality (and its 13 types), establishes distribution tables whose first overall analysis brings out a preponderance of witchcraft theories in Africa and in the Mediterranean basin, theories about aggression by Spirits in East Asia and the Pacific Islands, and those about sorcery in North and South America. If the gathering of facts is incontestably more systematic and the elaboration of interpretation less hasty with Murdock than with Foster, both bear out the difficulties of anthropology in exploiting the typologies which ought to serve as a departure point in its analyses.

Foster tries to pre-empt the objections which could be made against him. Certain illnesses caused by emotional disorders such as fear, shame and anger are difficult to classify rigorously and exclusively in the category of "personalistic" or "naturalistic", but it is the absence or presence of bad intentions or premeditation in the agents of illness to which Foster attributes inclusion in one or other category. Thus the *sustro* of Latin America, a fear caused by meeting a ghost or spirit, the *muina*, an anxiety also observed in Latin America where it is believed to be due to anger, which itself is a reflection and result of difficult interpersonal relations, the *chipil*, which in Mexico and Central America indicates apathy and manifestation of tiredness in a child whose mother is pregnant, seem to him more "naturalistic" than "personalistic": the first two are the result of a chance encounter and the third is not attributable to the will of the foetus.

Foster further remarks that the two types of etiology are often present in the same society, one or the other simply being predominant. Thus he can support his case with an article of Maria M. Suarez[8] based on the village of El Mororo in Venezuela — where 80% of the illnesses studied in the sample have a "natural" cause and only 11% a "supernatural" cause — to conclude that the system of causality in this group is "naturalistic", whereas Fortune's[9] observations on the Dobu of Melanesia ("Death is caused by witchcraft, sorcery, poisoning, suicide, or actual assault") moves him to think that causality of the "personalistic" type dominates there. Now Foster does not hide the fact that, in his opinion, "personalistic" theories are older that those about natural causality and he considers that in all fields, notably those about illness, the capacity to "depersonalise" causes constitutes progress in cultural evolution.

Independently of this last statement, which is hardly contestable in this form, Foster's line seems to invite certain criticisms which, over and beyond, can be aimed at the presuppositions and uncertainties of "medical" anthropology in general.

The voluntary action/involuntary action distinction (which permits the classification of Central and South American etiologies in the "naturalistic" type) has demonstrated its inadequacy in the debates on the relation between "witchcraft" and "sorcery". Let us remember that the action of the witch, opposed by Middleton and Winter[10] to that of the sorcerer due, notably, to its supposedly involuntarily character, is in fact, in the very idea which those who believe in its effectiveness have of it, very complex and ambiguous. Theories which make witchcraft an innate power define those who possess it as agents condemned to wish evil and perfectly given to choose their moment and, within the limits prescribed by the rules, their victim. The way in which power is acquired can itself only rarely be defined with any rigour as voluntary or involuntary. Between heredity and apprenticeship (two modalities which moreover are not always considered incompatible) numerous possibilities exist, from chance to error passing through negligence, which always makes the sorcerer a being partly responsible and partly victim of the acts which he commits, an individual will which is at the same time a structural outcome.

When Foster writes that the system of natural causality and the system of personal causality can coexist, he is only introducing within a particular culture his distinction between two types of illness characterised by the difference in their respective etiologies. But he is only putting back what he needlessly separated. Contrasting definitions of health and illness in terms of compatibility and incompatibility, of balance and imbalance between substances, humours or qualities are not contradictory with a persecutive conception of illness. It is not then simply a question of pointing out that two distinct systems of cause can apply to two corresponding series of illness but to observe that, to explain the same illness, within one society or one cultural unity, the role of the intellectual, symbolic relation between substances or qualities and that, also structural, of social agents are thought of as a continuity, according to one logical progression. Thus it is that in all societies of akan culture (Ashanti, Agni, the lagoon people of the Ivory Coast), one of the malevolent actions attributed to aggressive witchcraft consists in separating from each other two psychic instances whose strict congruence is necessary to the mental and psychic balance of the individual, to sustain as a consequence problems with vision, mental disturbances and, if a rapid end is not put to this split, death.

The distinction between one sector considered virtually as empirical-rational and one considered as irreducibly magical condemns one to ignore the problems of effectiveness and the real implications of the etiological system. Medical anthropology often tends to proceed with illness like Malinowski does with culture. When Malinowski,[11] in a table with three headings (which he subsequently complicates to account for a reality which he obviously has some difficulty in ordering), tries to get the survival of tradition and influences, the interest and intention of white people, and processes of cultural change and contact apart, Gluckman[12] observes that the table serves well in classifying the data, but in no way understanding it. For its part, medical anthropology realises a tour de force in classifying data independent of any cultural contact (even more so since it includes situations where Western influence plays a role) and, in so doing, making them to a large extent incomprehensible. In addition, it tends to project the division which it has created into local systems as if the social actors were at times scientific, at others magical, as if recourse to the "supernatural" meant for them an intellectual renunciation, as they resigned themselves, like good Christians, to separate knowledge from faith. On this one could observe that the renewal of interest in "traditional medicine" sometimes stems from a self-interested point of view in indigenous pharmacopoeia whose effective qualities the big pharmaceutical laboratories are very keen to pick up, whereas, from another side, a mystic interpretation of the particular gifts of exotic healers is developing, which itself would give rise to commercial exploitation (tourism, films, literature).

These strange avatars of ethnological enquiry and empiric/magical typology only indirectly concern our proposition. On the one hand they sanction in a certain way the elimination of the social dimension from illness which ought to interest the anthropologist as a matter of priority, on the other hand they flow more particularly from the interpretive system which the alternative terms empiric/magical make the object of a deliberate option of local thought. This interpretation is obvious with authors such as Eva Gillies[13] when she speaks of approaches "empiric in intention" or like V.W. Turner[14] himself when he suggests that it is possible that certain medicines are used by the Ndembu because they are "objectively effective". These authors intend to qualify claims according to which in certain societies any illness has a social cause. Consequently they attempt to demonstrate that certain illnesses, in the societies which they study, do not have a cause of this type (one will describe it, by opposition, as "natural") and that they are treated without a ritual process of divination, invocation or exorcism. Thus E. Gillies, concerning the village of Ogori in Nigeria, observes that certain illnesses, such as malaria, various fevers, hepatitis, gonorrhoea and Guinea worms, are the object of a "natural" explanation and treatment based on plants (in contrast with animal and human matter used in rituals intended to ward off or combat illnesses which have a magical explanation). Noting that Evans-Pritchard mentions with the Azande two childhood illnesses which are the only ones, to his knowledge, not to imply the action of sorcery or magic, she formulates the hypothesis that the oracles are not consulted about them and regrets that the author does not give more details about the causes which are attributable to them and the therapy which they involve. Information about the latter, she adds, "might have provided a clue to causal classification, since a non-magical medicine, empirically specific in intent, would seem to imply a naturalistic explanation for the disease" (p. 381).

Towards a restatement of the problem

It is clear that identification between the "magical" and the "social" results from the privilege given to the notion of cause, a privilege which is also found in the theme of the plurality of causes which Evans-Pritchard first developed to account for the fact that an illness whose fundamental cause is judged to be "social" can or must nevertheless be the object of physical treatment. This plurality of causes is particularly invoked in cases of accident to the body due to an immediately physical event (a branch or stone falling, etc). Now, there are social dimensions of illness other than etiological, dimensions properly intellectual which are not identified with the institutions of diagnostic and healing. The typological line neglects them and thus even prevents considering the whole social pattern which give their coherence and their effectiveness to nosology and therapeutic practice.

Moreover E. Gillies is very near making the same statement when, after having carried out a critical review of anthropological classifications and having suggested taking the symptomal diversity into consideration, taking an interest in the question "how?" and not simply in the question "who?", she remarks that, if Turner's work is one of the best there is on African medicine, it is because he was principally interested in "world views, symbols and underlying patterns of thought". But in maintaining the magic/empiric alternative at the centre of her thesis, she does not allow herself to explore the partly open trail, notably distinguishing a level of theoretic etiology (one where belief in witchcraft is manifest) and a level of the pathogenesis of common sense, which comes more or less back to reformulating the theory of the plurality of causes.

Now, it is quite surprising to observe that an author as well known and as often quoted as Erwin H. Ackerknecht had, from 1946,[15] strongly qualified the distinction which implicitly underlies the research bearing on "primitive medicine" and according to which "primitive medicine is primarily magico-religious, utilizing a few rational elements, while our medicine is predominantly rational and scientific employing a few magic elements". According to him, illnesses which ethnologists qualify as "natural" simply correspond to realities for which local populations have no explanation. These common pains are the object of traditional, mechanical treatment, about which no one cares to establish the overall theory: "To call such attitudes 'naturalistic' or 'rational' seems to inject into the data contents they actually do not have. People in this case operate below the threshold of full consciousness".

One could be surprised by the absence of reference to the notion of the unconscious for Ackerknecht and by his inability to answer to a question which the apparent heterogeneity of interpretations and therapies applied to the different symptoms of indisposition never ceases to bring up. In fact, the different medical techniques do not appear to invoke fundamentally contrary options to him: in many cases (notably with the Thonga described by Junod,[16] the Akamba studies by Lindbom[17]) the different specialists have different knowledge and roles but all share the reference to what Ackerknecht continues to call "the supernatural" with the ethnological tradition, the healer connoisseur of herbs is not different, in this respect, from the diviner. Professional specialisation cannot provide an argument for those who wish to distinguish a "rational" sector in primitive medicine at any price. Their mistake, according to Ackerknecht, comes essentially from the confusion which is established more or less implicitly with them between the "rational" and the "objectively effective". Thus an author such as Harley,[18] whom he considers to be one of the best observers of primitive medicine, does not differentiate under the term "rational", which he uses several times to analyse Mano therapy, between the notions of "logical", "effective" and "empiric". Ackerknecht denounces this confusion and the one which, linked to the fact that certain psychological mechanisms are the same in primitive and modern medicine, could lead the role of suggestion to be regarded with an equal eye in one and the other. Now, the suggestion of the shaman comes through a shared belief in the action of spirits, which is not the case with doctors. We will follow him up to a certain point in the claim of this distinction. It is quite obvious that there is a metaphoric dimension in the claim, for example, of the psycho-somatic character of certain African, medical practices. It is true that the content of belief can neither be abstracted from the study nor confused with the mechanisms of psychological effectiveness and that a notable, intellectual difference separates, even in these regions, traditional from modern medicine: "Ideational contents and psychological mechanisms are not the same phenomena..." (p. 161).

But one can also see that, on this last point, the difference in not as clear cut as certain claims would lead one to understand. Ackerknecht himself speaks of a difference of degree and not kind. He also evokes the supernatural element which exists in modern medicine, especially in patient expectation. For the rest, he clearly stresses the radical character of opposition between the two systems. According to him, the rational elements, which would be many in traditional medicine, would there themselves be completely integrated into an overall magical system. As for medical ignorance in modern societies, which could be as great as in primitive societies, it would concern natural fact, not spiritual influences or magical powers (except in the remotest countryside and certain particular sectors of cities). It is uncertain whether or not the author is sinning here through rationalist optimism. One knows the present day vogue for fortune tellers and clairvoyants of all sorts. But the conclusion of his article might appear more clearly disappointing on two important points.

In his legitimate anxiety to show that primitive medicine can more pertinently be defined as "logical" rather than "rational", he goes as far as opposing non-rational/rational (primitive medicine/modern medicine) the principal object of research in medical anthropology: "... The central problem lies in the differences between primitive and modern medicine. One of the essential aspects of this problem is how numerous rational (in the sense of empirical) elements are in primitive medicine and what role they play. The statement that primitive medicine is logical does not answer in any way this question" (p. 160). In a parallel way magic, reduced to the category of superstition, is defined as irrational without delving into the question of knowing in what way it can be logical. By ignoring the social character of this logic, the author reintroduces on one hand the dichotomy which he had put aside on the other and he gives a derisory character to the comparison between the two medicines which he however makes the prime object of anthropology. Contrary to the intentions demonstrated elsewhere,[19] he inscribes this comparison within an evolutionist perspective for which the supernatural and irrational elements to be found in modern societies appear as survivals. And it is these supernatural elements which he wishes to observe in their primary state, at the heart of primitive societies: "Even if I would accept J.M. Cooper's somewhat bold statement that primitive culture is 95 to 98 per cent purely rational and scientific, I would still place the bulk of primitive medicine among the remaining 2 to 5 per cent" (pp. 154–160).

Ackerknecht has the merit of emphasizing that there is, beyond technical specialisations, an ideological unity in traditional medicine, to suggest that rationality is not directly related to therapeutic effectiveness, to recognize that he does not measure traditional and modern medicine by the same yardstick. This last claim has its basis in its correspondence to a desire not to reduce primitive medicine to a few "rational" elements which permit its definition as a forerunner or mere sketch of our own. But it eliminates the question of knowing if the relation between medicine and society in traditional and modern societies cannot be examined from an entirely different point of view. The ambiguity, once again, comes from the uncertain use of the term "magic" which for Ackerknecht as for many others, either goes back to pure irrationality or else places the social under the sign of the supernatural or irrational because it applies before anything to an etiology. For all authors, one can speak of magic with primitive people and not with ourselves because illness with us is not social in the same way as with them.

We would like to ask ourselves here about the possibility of formulating a contrary proposition. It is only to the extent that illness is, in certain respects, equally social in various types of society that one can speak of it as an anthropologically significant phenomenon.

II. THE SOCIAL DIMENSION OF ILLNESS: THE EXAMPLE OF LINEAL SOCIETIES

A few preliminary remarks can be made in support of this claim:

First of all, it is not possible to suppose (which certain analyses of the empirical/magical alternative imply) that practicioners of traditional medicine either choose at certain moments to mock the results of their treatment or else operate a systematic distinction between organic illness and that stemming from psycho-somatism. However, only one of these two hypotheses would explain that they might have intentional recourse to non "objectively effective" treatments, to use Turner's terms. Now it is easy to see that, in terms of intentions, or in terms of results, things are not so clear. By definition ritual activity, for he who practises it, considers itself effective. The ancestor, the sorcerer who inherits his powers, the *vodu*, stomach-ache and animal sacrifice are no less "natural" than headache and medicinal herbs.[20] And if one judges by results, even without being as sceptical as Evans-Pritchard about local pharmacopoeias, one cannot exclude the possibility that the witch doctor supposed to see off the devourer of body and soul, might not be as effective as he who treats with plants and herbs. Moreover, in numerous cases, the same man treats the same illness with herbs and techniques of word, rite or spiritual force at the same time. Certain religions can be quite materialist in that the strength of their Gods is directly related to the charge of energy in their representations. Each *vodu* in Togo, in mina or ewe country, for example, has many representations. Thus Hevieso and Sapata are present in many courtyards and shrines and, one could say, totally present in each of their materialisations. Nevertheless, one can speak at each occurrence, in translation, of *a HEVIESO* or *a SAPATA*, of unequal strength according to whoever set them up and knows their internal formula (in the sense that one speaks of a chemical formula) being more or less competent, more or less abreast of the right combinations of elements, notably vegetable, which constitute the internal "charge" of each figure of the God — a charge which fades with use and which the initial installer must regularly renew.

Secondly, and more generally, there are no particular consequences to be drawn from the fact that traditional, nosological classifications more often order the causes of illness, or from the fact that these causes are for the most part conceived of as social. The history of Western medicine witnesses the difficulty that professional observers of illness have had in elaborating an ordering of its manifestations. Foucault has clearly shown in his *History of Madness in the Classical Age*,[21] in the chapter "The madman in the garden of species" that the positivist ideal — to classify according to visible signs — finds itself almost necessarily diverted towards a body of moral categories or towards a causal system. This detour — which has it that it is outside madness that one must seek the nature of madness — does not concern only madness. It is without doubt not attributable to a mere failure of thought or to inadequate scientific elaboration. After all, in certain sectors of modern therapeutics, it is admitted that the symptom not only is not the whole of the illness, but could moreover stem in principle from several possible causes, as if it was in some way the personal mark of illness, the originals monotone coloration which each individual complexion imprints on diverse, physiological causes. Conversely this does not preclude that a symptom might transpose itself without each of its manifestations stemming from a distinct cause. A mechanical, symptom-cause correspondence is therefore all the less easily conceivable since the symptom may be changing (or being transposed) without changing the cause. Such at least seems to be one of the hypotheses of psychosomatic medicine.

So, it is a statement of principle which makes many observers or analysts postulate a radical difference between the empirical interpretation of illness and their "social" or "magical" interpretation. Ackerknecht recognises the unique character of the framework of interpretation but underlines the "magical" that is to say "social" orientation of this framework. More subtly, or more usefully, Robin Horton[22] has tried to show, concerning Africa, that propositions which are on the principles of "magico-religious" systems are the same as those which underlie scientific systems. Let us remind ourselves, to raise here only the so-called social problem of etiology, the second of the propositions made by Horton: the distinguishing feature of theory is to place things in a broader causal context that provided by common sense. So for Horton there is no more sense in saying that a traditional African thinker is more interested in supernatural than natural causes than there would be to say that a physicist is more interested in atomic theory than natural causes. The broadening of causal context can be made in different directions but it proceeds from the same principle.

As for the possibly social character of the cause and, more widely, of certain etiological systems, one must above all remark that it does not constitute the only social dimension of illness. The procedures and analyses which have just been evoked have in common, beyond their limited or partial interest, the fact of not taking into consideration the entirety of social dimensions, and they disbar themselves in doing so from thinking anthropologically, in other words comparatively, about the notion of illness. These dimensions appear to us as a first approximation, to involve a triple logic: a logic of differences which orders some in relation to others, by means of equivalence of opposition, the symbols which serve to think of the social and constitute its intellectual framework; a logic of references which establishes the possible (and thinkable) relationship between this symbolical logic and the empirical social order; a logic of event, or chrono-logic, which submits the relationship of meaning constituted by the first two to the evidence of a relation of force unveiled by history. Because there is no other history than real history, because, by definition, the order of possibilities (differences and references) can hold no event as contingent, it cannot contradict the historical order (individual and social). This last appears very much like the expression of the first, but like a sometimes difficult, indirect expression, bringing into question the too mechanistic equations which, for example, systems of law establish. In as much as events must have meaning, in as much as no meaning can truly contradict another, one cannot conclude that meaning is deduced mechanically from event. In order for the system to hold, the surprises of history must translate its complexity, not its incoherences.

Let us go back to the "elemental" form of event which is illness. From the logic of differences come certain symptoms (hot, cold, sweat, dehydration...) or certain substances (blood, sperm, water, excrement...) which enter into the overall symbolic framework the elements of which manifest themselves in different sectors of social activity and in different practices or institutions, ritual or not. The binary oppositions which ethnologists have located in numerous "systems of thought" involve this logic of differences where, for example, heat opposes cold, like dry to damp. From this logic, one can doubtless say that, as an overall system, it is unconscious. It would be possible to show that, in this sense, the *pisa* illness found among the Alladian of the Ivory Coast entails the same logic as the forbidding of copulation on the ground in the bush. *Pisa* is the illness of the man who spits blood and weakens himself. The cause which one ordinarily attributes to it is the adultery of the wife; the equivalence blood = sperm, the warm character of blood-sperm and the principle of incompatibility of warm with warm explains, in symbolic terms, that the sperm of the man deceived by his wife cannot mix with or be added to that of her other sexual partner and flows back in the form of blood vomited or spat out. By the same token, the earth being warm, copulation on the ground entails on accumulation of warmth on warmth which incurs risks of dehydration and sterility.

Françoise Héritier[23] has shown the multiple and diversified aspects of the relationships between hot, cold, dry and wet in Samo representations and institutions in Upper Volta, notably from the point of view of the sexual differences and inequalities which these relationships give a shape. She also demonstrates that with the Samo, cold is associated with damp, warmth with dry, that the first connotes notion of prosperity, well-being and peace, the second that of danger. The master of rain, which is cold, is himself warm. A whole series of taboos and rites enter into the logic of relations, exclusions and compatibilities thus put in place. We will cite two particular expressions: blood is hot and, if the pregnant woman is particularly warm, it is that she is no longer loosing her blood and stores up that which, an avatar of sperm, comes to her from her husband to strengthen the child to be born. If childhood is a dangerous period it is because it corresponds to an accumulation of heat which only diminishes with the girl's first period and the boy's first emission of sperm ("the water of sex"). A sterile woman without periods, "an extreme example of all the cases of female sterility", accumulates blood and heat without ever losing them. Before burying her, her back is pierced at the kidneys to permit her to cool off and to prevent her heat, mixed with the earth's, from bringing on drought. The relationships thus illustrated in the Samo case seem to Françiose Héritier to broadly constitute a logic "of identity and difference" present, according to variable modalities, in all cultures.[24]

For many reasons (history, contact, forgetfulness) this logic, called logic of differences here, is not (or no longer) always comprehensible, even partially, in a coherent form. But illness, more precisely the analysis of symptoms, often offers one of the rare possible openings onto what can be glimpsed of it. The weakening of the logic of difference, from this point of view, can have two opposing consequences: either a relative degree of attention given to symptoms, but less focus on social etiology, or else a deficient symptomatology, but through the intermediary of divination, a considerable importance accorded to social and religious causes. Southern Togo, a region of migrations, covered long since by Gods of ones and others (Akan influence on one side, Yoruba and Fon influence on the other), a region where individual initiatives, which in this matter date right back, mix in the same place divinities of different origins "selected" by chance encounter or rumour, according to the idea that people had of their strength or the prestige of their "installer", provides good examples of this alternative.

In fact one finds here, side by side, two therapeutic systems which at first glance could be taken as exemplary representations of each of these two terms: the one of individual healers who take charge, through the intermediary of *vodu* and specific therapeutic and ritual procedures, of patients whose symptoms they have identified, the one of hereditary schools which recruit, according to precise social criteria, a certain number of initiates following illnesses or disease of very variable appearance, but whose cause and significance are identified through the divination of the oracle of Fa.

Quite naturally it is the individual healers, small entrepreneurs in therapeutic ideology who, welcoming a diverse clientele out of its usual, social context, formulate the most general diagnostics, elaborating a relatively narrow symptomatology. The logic of differences is only glimpsed in snatches and in a necessarily non-coherent way. The *vodu* healers are of diverse origins and, if they allow themselves to be ordered in relation to each other in the shrine where they gather, it is less as a function of their therapeutic specialisation (many of them are generalists) than as a function of taboos or attributes which, due to their tribulations, present themselves rather a heritage and historical chance. The diverse origins of patients, the fact that certain of them come from town, have as a consequence parallel with a lesser symbolisation of symptoms, an acute attention given to these, without the symbolic link uniting them to their social cause being very obvious.

As an example, we will briefly describe how things happen with one of the "independent" healers in Mina country, 'S', from the village of

Seko, near Anecho. 'S' introduces himself as a specialist healer (madness, asthma, heart troubles) who gives treatment by means of an apparently sophisticated pharmacopoeia. At the same time, he is a priest to two series of *vodu* grouped in two separate halls, whose intervention in healing is, according to him, decisive. The first altar is that of the *vodu* Agbe M'pa, of Ghanaian origin. Agbe M'pa is an "individual" *vodu*. He does not belong to a particular lineage within which his worship would be inherited. 'S' went to seek him in Bando, in Ghana, from a healer-priest of whom he had heard. To acquire a *vodu*, is on one hand to be initiated into it, to take recognition of the prescriptions and taboos which are attached to the practice of the cult, to learn the material composition of the God (whose statue is "charged" with herbs, minerals and other substances, the nature and relative proportions of which the profane world knows nothing), to thus acquire the quality of eventual re-installer of the *vodu* in question. On the other hand it is to pay, and possibly pay dearly, for the right of use of the *vodu* and thus carry out a symbolic and economic placement whose benefits will be measured by the success of the healer-priest who has just made the acquisition (acquiring, in some way, in medical terms, a new "speciality") and by the demand for installation which will possibly be addressed to him. The installation must be made by the previous holder of the *vodu*. So 'S' had, apart from everything else, to pay the costs of travel and board of the Ghanaian priest of Agbe M'pa, who had come to Seko, "to start on its journey" the copy which conformed to the original model, whose formula had been delivered to him in Ghana. Of course, one cannot handle such powers with impunity, and 'S' could justly point out that he was already familiar with the *vodu* and healing before setting up his own altars and starting his own business.

Agbe M'pa is used (this term can surely be employed, as Gods in the situation give the impression of being controlled by men) in private affairs, notably matrimonial, matters of sport (disputes between rival clubs, offensive and defensive preparations for sporting contests) and in cases of madness. The shrine where he is to be found contains quite a large number of figures of other minor *vodu* grouped around what one might call the central theme, the theme of bi-sexuality represented by a seated couple. The man and woman have red faces. A red handled knife rests in the woman's hands. The man, who is wearing a necklace made of small bottles around his neck, brandishes a knife handle in his right hand. Between his feet an object seeming to depict a couple facing each others bound by tightly tied ropes, describes the central theme on a smaller scale. To the right of the man several statuettes (one in white clay, two in red wood covered with raffia skirts) symbolize the association of the altar of Agbe M'pa with tobacco and smoke. Cigarettes have been slipped into the holes which represent the mouth. One can smoke beside Agbe M'pa's altar and offer him tobacco. The *vodu* also accepts alcohol. Firstly the priest drinks his feminine representation, then his masculine representation. Next he pours a little alcohol on different objects, among which the bound couple between the feet of the masculine *vodu*. Red oil (palm oil) is the *vodu*'s absolute taboo.

The second altar is that of Madi Lasa, which comes from neighbouring Benin (Dahomey). The altar is in fact made by the elaborate reunion of a multitude of minor altars of *vodu* who can be considered as messengers or go between who speak to Lasa. All the *vodu* of this chapel accept red oil (palm oil) as well as alcohol. This difference with Agbe M'pa is a more general one (distinguishing between "oil" *vodu* and *vodu* "without oil"). This hits you immediately if you visit the two types of altar one after another. The oil altars are places of numberless libations. Under the layer born of the accumulation of coagulated blood and oil, the shape of the statues can just be made out, as if they were the result, not of the building up of solid matter, but rather the gradual melting of some immense block of wax. Lasa will bear neither tobacco nor smoke. Several statues at the altar are covered in chains to which padlocks have been attached. According to an explanation immediately provided by 'S' these padlocks "attach" the requests which are made to him to the *vodu*. They are locked by the petitioner, who will unlock them once satisfaction has been obtained. But it seems probable that the meaning attached to this licking might be less defensive or less innocent. *Aze*, the aggressive power of the sorcerer, is also just that which enables attack by witchcraft to be warded off. In Guin and Mina country there is a theory of witchcraft. It is supposed to transmit itself preferentially through the maternal line, to be able to act on the socially or geographically nearest, neighbours or relatives, but under any conditions (a son can kill his father, but not a father his son, conversely a woman can kill her children, but they can do nothing against their mother). Thanks to intermediaries, an aggressor can however reach someone who is not related to him and lives far from him. The interesting, thing is that, contrary to what happens elsewhere and for example at present with the lagoon people of the Ivory Coast, the *aze* system is well integrated into that of *vodu*. There are *aze vodu* whose worship can obviously not be practised by just anyone, complete mastery of the cult being on the contrary the object of initiation by stages and the *aze*, generally, can only be manipulated, repelled or attacked by those who possess it. We have described at greater length elsewhere[25] the case of the Akpaso *vodu* which is used to attack as well as defend. Spiritual power, manipulative practice and ritual activity are associated in the struggles of which *aze* is the stake, means or object. That their presence might be kept more secret, the *aze vodu* are often present at the side of others in sanctuaries run by the individual entrepreneurs of ritual therapy. The distinctions witchcraft/sorcery, religion/magic, witch/witch doctor do not entirely account for this kind of figure.

The *aze vodu* accept and appreciate red oil and eggs. So they are logically present in 'S''s second shrine. The two shrines oppose each other symbolically, even if they complement each other as regards to practice, in relation to a certain number of criteria. In the first there are *vodu* who like tobacco and smoke to whom red oil is forbidden. They are from Ghana and receive mostly vegetable offerings. Alcohol is common to both shrines, but tobacco and oil exclude each other. In the second shrine, the *vodu* from Dahomey who like red oil receive mostly animal and egg offerings. The red oil-eggs-chains and padlocks association is witnessed in other altars where there are *aze vodu*. Agbe M'pa is bisexual, Lasa is feminine.

All these oppositions do not immediately make sense. Moreover, certain of them are relative (for example, the distinction between vegetable offerings and animal offerings does not absolutely cover the two altars). They do not seem to have an immediate parallel in the symbolism of the lineage and village (shrine) cults. Once again, the diversity of geographical and cultural origins of the gods and the patients would explain the rather truncated, or not easily perceptible, aspect of the logic of differences. Nevertheless, this diversity must itself be seen in proportion. On the one hand there is no irremediable divide between cultures of Akan type and cultures of Benin regions. On the other hand the latter (be it only a question of exchanges of all kinds carried out during the course of their history) have many common features. If someone such as Roberto Pazzi could put together a large body of work[26] — *eve, aja, gen, fon* — *et son univers*, it is because the words and notions which they evoke are very similar from one group to another. A piece of research of this kind brings out numerous points, aside from contrasts and correspondences which manifest themselves, within the diversity of individual institutions and practices, a common symbolism.

Thus the human body is the object of a very homogeneous representation which one sees in action in the practice of unction. The head is the reservoir of thought which rises from the back. In the head thought becomes action. The heart symbolizes and guarantees, like the drum in dance, the harmony between these two pokes. The stomach is the seat of feelings. The diviner who attributes the psychical or psychological troubles of a person to an insufficiency in the head or the back, these two vital poles, can direct him to make a sacrificial offering (asa) to his back or his head. As for the unctions they are applied to very precise places; the head at three cardinal points — forehead = east, head = zenith, nape = west, the heart, the middle of the back at the point corresponding to the central vertebra (Tu) which is the radial centre of bodily movement, the fold of the elbow and the knees, the thumbs and the toes (more exactly the big toe (afosu, the male of the foot) which is supposed to control the others and express the autonomy of the person (Pazzi, pp. 145 and 179). Pazzi further remarks that in these diverse cultures, the conception of the human organism does not only express itself in rites but also in a language which is "structured on suffixes which derive from its different members". Thus "against" is said as "body", "above" "head", "in front of" "mouth", "beside" "ear", etc.

We find this conception of the body at work in the practice of individual priest-therapists, and more precisely in the treatment by unction of certain forms of madness. In the same way, the equation red oil = blood, witnessed in the Aja, Fon, Guin or Ewe cults (Pazzi, p. 96) is obvious to any onlooker at the second of 'S's altars. In the same way again, the distinction between warm leaves (*Ama dzodzo* in Ewe, *ama zozo* in Aja Guin and Fon) and cold leaves (*ama fafa* in Ewe, Aja, Guin, *ama fifi* in Fon) applies to all: the first dry, disperse malevolent influences and enliven the body and will power, the latter re-establish the calm and balance of the organism. The care, potions, bathing and internal composition of the *vodu* involve the same categorisation, just as much as the various forms of incantation which aim to influence the Gods, to attack men or to defend oneself from them. Incantation is called *"amagbe"* (*"voice of the leaves"*).

Overall however, the thing which strikes one with individual therapists is the sharpness of the symptomatology, especially in fields where it seems clear that, traditionally, it was absent, and the broad character (one could say historical or sociological rather than social) of the etiology. Let us return to 'S'. He described to us with a certain number of details the diverse sorts of madness which he has to treat. Traditionally, madness was not really named, but alluded to indirectly: *Tadu* ("the head has bitten") in Fon, *adahwa* ("the hair is wet") in Guin (Pazzi, p. 150). Moreover it is just this term which 'S' uses. But madness is such a mysterious illness that, when it resisted the administration of very strong, tranquillising plants, society saw only two possible solutions: aggressive and dangerous, the madman was done away with; inoffensive, he was allowed to wander freely, but naked, so that, no one risked being deceived. 'S' claims to heal these madmen.

He distinguishes several types of madness, according to the patient's manifestations and at the same time in relation to the cause that they invoke. In a first category are ranged all the types of madness brought about by the *vodu* themselves (*vodu* from the paternal or maternal lines which demand reinstatement in the family which has neglected them or attacks of witchcraft inflicted through specialised *vodu*). In the case of a demand to return, in other words the installation of an altar, the patient stays laid low and in bed at home. He refuses to speak until the moment when he cries out that he is pursued by a *vodu*. The man who is sick due to a *vodu* is more wretched and depressed than other patients. Some have been brought to 'S' after a suicide attempt. This is the only case which demands, for confirmation and clarification of the identity of the *vodu*, a consultation of divination by Fa (there is a Fa priest at Seko). It is the latter who gets closest to the diagnosis after which a man or a woman enters a shrine.

The second form of madness would be due to a worm, *koko*, probably introduced into the body through aggressive witchcraft. It manifests itself through a mild agitation (the mad person is not restrained: he does not speak much, shouts from time to time, sings to himself endlessly) but also by precise physiological symptoms a kind of pus comes out of the eyes and anus.

Madness due to drugs (Indian hemp or marijuana) gives rise to the most violent manifestations. The madman can only be transported to Seko chained and bound. Once there he might have to be chained up. On his arrival, he cannot sleep, even after being given a sleeping draught.

The madness "of religion" demonstrated that the *vodu* (and their priests) are very attentive to the rise of white, Christian syncretisms. Pentacostalists, Jehovah Witnesses, members of Alladura or Cherubim sects are considered as sworn enemies by the *vodu* priests. The member of the new sects is rejecting the *vodu*, is spurning the taboos attached to its situation, but, insufficiently strong, he is attacked by his *vodu*. Less agitated than the drug takers, he claims not to be ill, but he feels threatened and persecuted by everybody. Men and the *vodu* want to kill him, he thinks, and he expresses his anxiety in endless speeches.

Two last kinds of madness are, in some ways, the backlash of an imprudent manipulation of *vodu* forces, of an individual's over-estimation of his own strength and an under-estimation of another's. One does not invoke with impunity the *aze vodu*. One does not tempt fate against

someone with impunity. In both cases, one must be equal to the forces
that one is using or confronting.

All these types of madness are not cared for in the same way, whereas
certain treatments (notably sleep treatment after taking a tranquillising
infusion based on "cold" leaves, *ama fafa*) are common to both. In the case
of madness due to drugs, one has seen, it is difficult to get the patient to
sleep (it is even one of the distinctive signs of this ailment). After having
made him drink the tranquillising infusion, a few incisions are made on
him onto which is spread a little black powder obtained by pounding
cold herbs, part of the composition of Agbe M'pa, the *vodu* who likes
smoke. This treatment has the explicit goal of "diminishing his strength".
After twenty four hours, the treatment is repeated, which, finally, produces an effect. On wakening (after one or two hours), he generally
admits to having smoked "hemp", and this admission confirms the
diagnostic, but not necessarily the cure. The cure, which would last from
three to eight months — depending, says 'S' on the lapse of time between
the start of the illness and the moment when the patient was taken to
him — involves putting drops into the eyes, ears and nose, and inhala-
tions. In each case the liquid used contains herbs of Agbe M'pa, as does
the "soap" that the patient uses to wash. Everyday, palmist oil is rubbed
on the patient's body, white and not red like palm oil. The oil palm (Elaeis
guineensis) in fact provides, it is known, two sorts of oil: palm oil,
obtained from the pulp of the fruit, and palmist oil, extract of almond.
As for the food taboos which define the patient's "diet" they do not
absolutely discriminate since they also concern tobacco and alcohol, as
well as red meat, red oil, pork, gumbo, fresh fish and vegetables.

In the case of the madness of "religion", after first passing before Agbe
M'pa, to whom the priest explains the case, the patient is immediately
led before Oasa and anointed with red oil. Next relatives wash him with
water containing herbs of this *vodu* (picked in Benin). The influence sends
him to sleep very quickly. When he reawakens, he recites prayers or
sings hymns of his sect, thus confirming the diagnostic established after
the first symptoms. The care which is given to him is of the same kind
as that given to drug takers, but the herbs are those of Lasa, as in the case
of those whom a neglected *vodu* has made mad. In both cases, it is the
reappearance of speech (a calmed speech) which bears witness to the
cure. The cured patient stays for some time with 'S' and so serves as
helper and intermediary for others.

In 'S''s view, therapeutic failure is impossible. Certainly there are
cured patients who have relapses. It is because they have not respected
the taboos, notably concerning diet (tobacco, alcohol, pork), or else they

have committed new errors. In sum, one can see that the identification of symptoms (we are not here concerned with comparing it with psychiatric nosologies, although certain descriptions invite it) entails the evocation of a certain number of problems linked to phenomena of acculturation: the resistance to change directly or indirectly imputable to Western influence is without doubt due to the efforts of free, therapeutic-religious enterprise.

A perceptible, but truncated, logic of difference, a fixed and precise symptomatology, and, from a sociological point of view, a fairly global etiology, therefore seem to go hand in hand with individual, therapeutic-religious enterprise. Behind the demands of his patients (or those of their entourage), 'S' feels or perceives a weakening of non-Christian religious patterns or at least, their effectiveness. The weakness of those who try for power, when they have neither power nor knowledge, leads them to try to manipulate forces which they do not know how to control, to neglect or to provoke Gods, whose power they have forgotten, and to abandon themselves to the temptations of drugs or sects. One could, in parenthesis, suggest concerning this last opinion that, if white syncretisms are so poorly regarded by *vodu* priests, whereas Catholicism and Protestantism as such leave them indifferent, it is because syncretic priest and *vodu* priests, to a certain extent, have the same goals, ascribe the same immediate end to their practices and see the effect of their practice whatever the outcome of events. They confront each other on the same ground.

	Agbe M'p a	*Lasa*
Symbols	smoke plants tobacco bisexuality	red oil = blood animals eggs (witchcraft) femininity
Illness	madness due to the use of drugs	madness due to the invocation or vengeance of *vodu*
Cures	palmist oil cold leaves (calm)	palm oil warm leaves (attack)
Origin	Ghana	Benin

The system of hereditary shrines, such as one can observe at the moment (still from the point of view of a weakening or fading of the logic of differences) offers a different, and almost opposite image of that of private altars. Illness is the source of the creation, divine presence and human recruitment of hospices, but it is not the symptom itself which directly signifies the requirement or call of the God. There must be an intermediary stage of divination (Afa, Fa) to which one has recourse whether due to the repetition of a biological trouble whose forms are not pre-defined, or whether due to the structural position of patients (for example young girls belonging to a line whose shrine is important) which designates them as more particularly exposed to the attention of the Gods.

We will take for example a shrine in the village of Anfouin. In the four quarters of the village there are numerous shrines (twenty three in 1974, but the process of creation goes on uninterrupted and two new shrines had just been founded in Anfouin in 1977 when I passed through again). Several priests can coexist in each of these shrines and several *vodu*, or several representations of the same *vodu*. Once his priest is dead, the worship of a *vodu* is charged to a member of his *Kota* (patrilineage). But a succession of events or illnesses can bring about the entry of new *vodu* into the shrine.

The shrine of the priest Kowuvi is situated in the Afeto home district (or rather just off it, for, due to the narrowness of this central district, where the chief resides, certain lineages have had to install their shrines in neighbouring districts, as it happens Kpodji, which can spread without hindrance towards the exterior). This shrine contains three Hevieso. Hevieso is an important God whose weapon and symbol is lightning. Pierre Verger[27] has observed that, in Abomey, two groups of *vodun* of very different character constituted Hevieso (whom the Fon call Hevioso): "A first group of Gods of thunder or *vodun* whose judgemental action is to cause death and destruction by lightning is found there side by side with another group of Gods whose activity is connected with sea and water" (p. 525). Pazzi describes this link and observes that, in conjunction with Lightning, the Sea is also venerated, under the names, in Guin, of Agbwe and Avlekete: "When the lightning becomes aroused, he comments, the Sea intervenes to calm this ardour". In fact, their complementary nature was subtler, as one can observe concerning the case of epidemic. Then all the *vodu* were mobilised to chase away the evil, however certain of them saw a particular role attributed to them, whether after a consultation with Fa, whether due to their specific attributes. Thus Hevieso and the other God of lightning, Sovi, were more specifically invoked to fight against smallpox of which Sapata is at the same time the cause, the symbol and the remedy. But it was the priestesses of Avlekete, whose "inverted" behaviour has been analysed elsewhere,[25] who intervened as a last resort. They were the last to dance and offer Sapata the food which was normally forbidden to him. For some Avlekete and Agbwe are "like twins" and they are the two wives of Hevieso but the Agbwese, contrary to the Avleketesi, do not display inversion-provocation behaviour. For others it is Avlekete and Agbwe who are "man and wife", but Agbwe also passes for the wife of Hevieso. For the Ewe of Be, in Lome, Agbwe is the feminine (and maritime) version of Hevieso or So, but it is the Agbwesi who display institutionally inverse or caricatural behaviour in respect of So and his initiates. These variations do not seem due to uncertainties of memory or to some historical erosion. P. Verger describes similar variations in the chapter which he devotes to the marine *vodun* of the Hula or Pla. In the Abomey region Burton[28] describes the masculine character of Avrekete. For Le Herissé,[29] Avrekete is the son of Agbe (Agbwe) also called Hou who is masculine. For Herskovits,[30] Afrekete is the daughter of Agbe who is himself the son of Sogbo, one of lightning *vodun* who make up Hevieso. In all, one finds in the Anfouin region an opposition-complementarity of the same type between a marine principle and a celestial principle, one more clearly marked by a feminine sign, the other by a masculine (the relative character of this opposition being due to the very generally bi-sexual character of the great divinities). Hevieso is indeed the God of lightning, the God of justice who strikes thieves (the dead by lightning, just as the dead by drowning, are the "bad dead"). For the rest, his relation to human illness is not specific. It is the consultation of Fa which uncovers in the illness of his future priests a recall to order and in the illness of his future initiates a call and a choice. The illness of the future priest appears in effect, after consultation of the oracle, like the reminder by a determined *vodu* of past negligence. Thus the *vodu* Hevieso, whose present priest is Kowuvi had first of all been discovered and, for an initial time, neglected by his great grandfather Kuevidze. The lightning stones (*Sokpe*) are meteorites or neolithic tools that are kept in the shrines of the Gods of lightning (Sogbo, Sovi, Hevieso). They are supposed to strike the victims of the latter and the ground is searched at the spot where a man has been struck by lightning or a hut set ablaze by lightning to find them. There are signs and, to some extent, materialisations of these Gods, more particularly Hevieso. The farmer who finds one in his field and brings it back home without identifying it, runs the risk of attracting the God's anger whose second recourse will take the form of illness. Now the stones are in general a sign of happiness and luck. A man who finds a beautiful stone might be tempted to take it without recognising the divine sign. Certain lightning stones are very easily identifiable, but stones of less common shape or piece of iron after the event (after the illness and the consultation of Fa) are less obvious divine objects. Kuevidze had found a large, strangely shaped stone. He took it back home with him. Later an illness obliged him to consult the Fa oracle. The latter revealed the identity and the request of the God to whom an altar and a shrine were immediately dedicated by the line. A rough calculation permits one to estimate the duration of this cult of lineage at around a century and a half. Six priests have taken charge of it: Kuevidze himself, Trenu, Kuevi Gbeke, Kodzovi, Voduivi (a woman) and Kowuvi, the present priest, who is also chief of all the Anfouin priests and therefore, in principle, in charge of the most ancient altar.

The succession to the priestly charge is made within the lineage, but it is subject to the consultation of Fa. A woman can be designated as well as a man, but the priests responsible for an altar are for the most part male. The inauguration ceremony lasts seven days and involves the whole village. It brings in the chief of the village priests, the holder of the most ancient altar.

It is a woman, a former follower, who most directly has charge of the

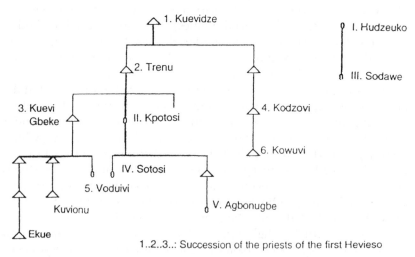

1..2..3..: Succession of the priests of the first Hevieso

I..II..III..: Succession of the Notu

shrine's female, initiate inmates (in the Anfouin region, there are no male initiate inmates). She can get help from female initiates like herself and whom she can choose. But she herself is designated by the priest according to her personal qualities, without consulting Fa (she has already been chosen by the God at the time of her initiation), most often within the priest's patrilineage. This woman bears the name *Notu* which is specific to Hevieso (for example the corresponding title is *Azana* or *Azrokpe* for the Agbwe *vodu*).

In the Kowuvi shrine, the memory is kept of five *Notu* who have had charge of the female initiates. The first of them was not from the same lineage as Kuevidze, but she was from the same district and had been part of the first intake of female initiates before becoming a *notu*, without doubt many years after the inauguration of the shrine. It is not known who carried out this role in the intervening time. In Anfouin, tradition has it that only women are initiated. This custom is not Guin, but local. In the next village to Aklakou, men spend a period of reclusion and initiation in the shrines. This period, which varies according to the Gods to which the initiates are dedicating themselves, is, in Anfouin, seven months in the shrines of Hevieso. So the *notu* assists the priest to initiate them into the rituals proper to this God and teaches them his language (each *vodu* generally has his own language), but the first task of the *notu* and the priest who knows Hevieso's herbs was to heal the inmates whose choice the illness has commanded. Exceptionally it can happen that some of them are voluntary, but in fact most of the *vodusi* enter the shrine following illness. The consultation of Fa then reveals either that a particular *vodu* has thus expressed his choice (a possession by the *vodu* will confirm to oracle's diagnostic), or either that a deceased, former initiate has been partially reincarnated and, at any rate, manifested in the person of the new one. This last type of succession can unite a paternal aunt to her niece or a mother to her daughter, in other words, the inmates or in general either daughters of the priest's patrilineage, the connection thus tending to be reinforced in symbolic terms in relation to the alliance, or else daughters of the latter, therefore from different *kota*. The designation by ancestor or by the Gods is quite restricting, when the chosen woman is married, to impose on her recalcitrant husband. Conflicts can arise on this occasion between in-laws and son-in-law, they easily being able to reproach him for putting the life of his wife in danger. Relationships of alliance can be put under a strain after this period of initiation (seven months of reclusion for Hevieso in Anfouin, during which the wearing of a white, cotton loincloth is obligatory, then an intermediary period which, depending on the wealth of the parents — for the second coming out ritual is expensive — can vary from a few days to three years and during which the female initiate live in the village, but wear the white loincloth and speak the language of the *vodu*. Finally, after the ritual which gives permission to wear an ordinary loincloth, four months lead to the final, coming out ritual, *gbehoho*, after which the concerned party can freely use everyday language). If the husband refuses to bear all the costs involved in the various ceremonies the father is free to remarry her to whoever will pay them off. Thus the costs of the cult, when they are incurred before the marriage of the young initiate, act a little like a dowry, a dowry paid to the *vodu* to whom the initiate's father is only the intermediary, which bears witness to the fact that, if he does not take back his daughter while refusing to be reimbursed by his son-in-law, the latter runs the risk, if he falls ill, of seeing his illness interpreted as a vengeance of the *vodu*.

Thus the shrines are an eminently social system, and regularly bring back to the village the daughters of the *kota* and the daughters of their daughters, a centripetal system in a world of intense mobility, system where one can well see that the diviner (bokono) plays an essential role. This is not the place to broach a subject which has been abundantly treated by Albert Néron de Surgy. Let us simply remind ourselves that one becomes a diviner following a long initiation, that following his apprenticeship the diviner installs in his home the *vodu* which the Oracle has prescribed to him (he is also a priest like the others), that the diviner as well has been "chosen" — the Oracle (*Afa*) having given him some psychologic or somatic trouble to invite him to reveal his choice through him — that if men and women can equally be diviners, the latter can only practise after menopause. As for the technique of divination by manipulation of sacred nuts and the deciphering of shapes obtained from a framework of sixteen squares, it shows that the symptom as such is not at the source of interpretation. This observation is equally valid for priests as for initiates and one can bear back pain, fever, stomach pains, fainting fits or eye trouble equally cited as signs of a call by the *vodu* to set up an altar to him or go back into his service.

The second Hevieso of Kowuvi's shrine is Ekue who is his grand nephew in agnatic line. Just over twenty years ago, Ekue, who was making drills for a yam plantation, had uncovered a semi-circular stone which resembled a man's face. At first he had kept it without saying anything. Another day, his uncle Kuvionu, who was working with him, uncovered lightning stones (*sokpe*) in the same place. The lightning stones could be taken as forming the *vodu*'s belt. When consulted, Fa revealed that it involved Hevieso and asked Kowuvi to set him up for Ekue. This inauguration dates from just after 1970, just as that of the third Hevieso. The story of this one is twenty years old. Guyo, a descendant of a former "foreigner" (slave?) from the village, had discovered in present day Ghana an impressive stone. His nephew, a *bokono*, revealed its therapeutic powers to him, when having returned to Anfouin, he showed it to him. Guyo enjoyed a reputation as a healer there (back pain), but he fell ill. The oracle, consulted after some time, demanded the setting up of a Hevieso, but Guyo died (he had waited too long, it was said) and, after a new consultation, it was Afanou who set up the new altar to Hevieso in 1973. None of these Hevieso are distinguishable by nosological attributes or specific, therapeutic powers, but the three recruit an imposing number of inmates (18 in 1977). The shrine and "convent" of Kowuvi, chief of Anfouin's priests, is one of the most important, but one can see that, overall, the system of shrines functions like a great, educative machine, which each year "treats" a relatively large number of young girls and women. From the therapeutic point of view the problems which precede recruitment are in general slight. The shrines, from this point of view, constitute an instrument for general medicine. More priest than doctor, the *hunõ* is above all the guarantor of the social and community sense of the event. The succession to the priesthood bears witness to this as well as the modalities of the recruitment of inmates. One can see in the pattern representing the succession to the charge of priest of Hevieso in Kowuvi's shrine that two lines of descent from Kuevidze represent an effort to maintain the cohesion of the lineage and avoid segmentation. This effort is quite conscious so that Kowuvi, anticipating moreover the oracle of Fa in an unorthodox way, has already designated Ekue, priest of the second Hevieso, as successor in charge of the main altar.

III. CLOSED COHERENCE, VIRTUAL COHERENCE

The logic of references is that which refers any biological disorder to a social disorder. We have just seen that it is difficult to invoke the logic of difference without bringing in at the same time the references which it implies (*pisa*, adultery and earth are taken within the same symbolic framework of warmth and blood, the respective roles of symptomatology, symbolism and social etiology, historically seem to be a function one of another). One and the other logics are rather distinct dimensions of a same logic, as is "chrono-logic", and one can try to delimit this identity from a certain number of observations.

Doubtless there are in numerous societies ills which are not mechanically explained by a cause of a social type. But neither symptomatology nor therapeutics radically distinguish these ills from others. In fact it is often the persistence of the pain, rather than its form, which elicits the hypothesis of a social cause, for example aggressive witchcraft. Many authors have noted it, but it must at the same time be observed that no discontinuity appears between pains with vague, but brief symptoms, pains with vague, but insistent symptoms, pains with precise symptoms for which there exists pre-determined etiology, but whose interpretation remains definitively linked to evolution over time. There is the same continuity in diagnostics and therapeutics. If, in these cases, there exists an etiological categorisation of vague or precise symptoms (aggression by witchcraft in the case of slow death, a paternal curse in the case of sudden death, adultery in the case of coughing blood, friction between parents in the case of a child's diarrhoea, among the Alladian), one must also be very clear on the one hand that such and such a social interpretation often involves a symbolism which comes directly from the logic of differences, on the other hand that the "medicine" used to treat ills with a "social" origin can purely and simply be plant substances which certain authors by definition place within the arsenal of empiricist and naturalist medicine. Thus among the Alladian each individual is born under one of three signs (water, forest, the dead) which also serve to distinguish categories of supposedly, supernatural agents and real healers. Taboos, possibly a special name, sanctioned to which of these signs one belonged. To the sign of the dead were linked clairvoyance and, more precisely, the art of uncovering the social causes (witchcraft) of illness, to the sign of the forest were linked the knowledge of plants and, more precisely, of therapeutic plants. The opposition between water and forest, which quite logically orders certain dimensions of Alladian society — and entails its division into two patrilineal halfs, distinguished by their birth rites — is therefore found in the domain of clairvoyance and healing. Water in fact constitutes a particularly and eminently ambiguous domain which confers great powers and exposes one to great risks. Madness is at the same time the speciality of water healers (*sekebo*) and that by which they are threatened. Death by drowning is a bad death but he who, finding the dead person's body, carries out the funeral rite in place of that person's relatives, will at the same time assure himself of many descendants. At the symbolic level therefore water is associated in a doubly ambiguous way with madness and life. Each of these poles in their turn divides up. Water cures madness and causes it. Drowning, the crowning of death or, in some sense, a double death which separates the victim from the village of the dead, from life after death and from eventual reincarnation, can also be a source of fertility for he who knows how to palliate its effects. The forest, in this light, is opposed to the water. It constitutes a threat to children, who are sometimes carried off by dwarfs, spirits of the forest. The forest and the dead are often associated, witness the breadth of power of certain *sekebo* who, embodying both at once, are capable of discovering social causes and of administering plant remedies. The amalgam water/dead is not attested to.

The symbolic elements which enter into the logic of differences in the form of equations or incompatibilities of the type blood/sperm, earth/blood, warmth/warmth, etc. also come into the logic of references, but they introduce the principle of discrimination which relativises the mechanistic aspect of the first. Blood is not evoked in its full physiological and symbolic reality as long as one does not speak about its transmission. Now, according to the modalities which can vary from one society to another, the transmission of blood is always conceived of as differential. The strongest blood is transmitted, with psychic principles and the powers which are associated with it, according to certain lines. There again, it is a question of a "theory" which has only retrospective value. In the light of events a younger could be revealed as stronger than an elder, have an accusation of witchcraft fall upon him or accede to the headship of the line. But the departure from the normal order does not call into question the principle of this order. One could say as much of all the psychic elements of the person or of the giving of a name. By definition, individuals are not equal or alike and these social differences are inscribed in their genetico-symbolic patrimony. This proposition, which will enchant the followers of socio-biology and the new right, is certainly the principle implicit in many lineal societies and it makes itself explicit on numerous occasions. But, used pragmatically, meticulously and retrospectively, it constitutes less a political and ethical principle than a principle of explanation of event, a way of using concrete history. The sum of the logic of differences and the logic of references notably constitutes the intellectual framework of social etiology. As this can give rise to the confrontation of social groups and certain symptoms are socially intelligible, the possibility exists (and is often manifest) of a split between relationships of meaning (symbolic) and relationships of force (social). The machinery of institutions applies itself to making good this, quite literally unthinkable, split, as needs be (it is the retrospective aspect of the theory) by diagnostic revisions. When all is said and done, the result is that the restriction linked to the logic of events simplifies the problems which it might seem to complicate.

Where illnesses have a diachronic dimension, events happen. The meaning of the illness is no longer simply read on the patient's body but possibly on that of others, of the surrounding company, of those who, in their turn, are born, dream, fall ill or die. As a rule, the logic of events or chrono-logic (the term "logic" only being justified by the supposed non-contingent character of the event) sanctions or confirms the relationship of force. But it expresses a dependence in respect of event that the social structure is sometimes not strong enough to eliminate. Symbolic effectiveness needs effectiveness pure and simple. The diagnostic demands the caution of the event. But, if death is always, from this point of view, the ultimate defeat of partners in the social game, it is good for the others to think about, which means that as a general rule and in the end, the relations of intra or interlineal force are not set in contradiction to the relations of meanings borne of the diagnostic of the illness or of the interpretation of the death.

The two examples which we have just developed allow us to delimit a little more precisely still what must be understood by the social dimension of illness. If the latter cannot be reduced to a causal dimension, it is because the order of differences functions in respect of particular interpretations and of the overall system of interpretation whose social etiology takes its place like a *principle of coherence*. The principle of coherence overflows the notion of causality but it is its foundation. The event/principle relation of coherence is often easily seen as a causal link, but neither always nor exclusively. The social references, one has seen, involve a symbolism of the same kind as that which commands the "natural" relations between warm and cold, dry and wet, etc. Illness with a social etiology and illnesses with a non-social etiology stem from the disturbed "social" or "natural" relationship, which explains the appearance within the same logic of differences functioning as a principle of coherence.

This principle of coherence, which forbids the radical opposition of two types of illness, explains certain apparent paradoxes. Thus it is not contradictory that an illness demands two types of treatment at the same time: a social treatment (the re-establishment of a normal, social relationship through admission, fine, sacrifice...) and an objectively vegetal treatment administered to the suffering body. It is no more unthinkable that, as one Alladian informer put it, there might be "more than one cause of the death of a man". The double causality scheme described by Evans-Pritchard is not exclusive to the coherence of principle which the

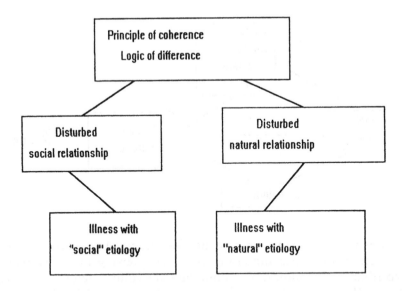

system supposes. Social etiology and "natural" etiology are not incompatible. In the same way, the revisions of diagnosis which frequently sanction the autonomous evolution of the symptom and the competition of social groups involved, the chronological dynamics, never allow the system as such to be doubted because the causal level is not the final authority. After all, there is nothing surprising in the split which can possibly introduce itself between the interpretative scheme and the therapeutic procedure. The latter can stem directly from the principle of coherence without passing through the mediation of cause.

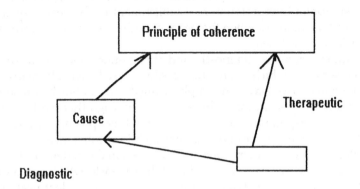

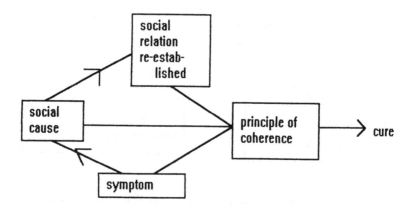

More widely, one can conceive that the interpretative procedure and the therapeutic procedure are more or less convergent or divergent according to the cultures or, within the same culture, according to the illness. Thus we can distinguish a closed coherence model and a virtual coherence model.

The closed coherence model corresponds to the ideal-type of interpretation in terms of social etiology: the symptom is classified by definition as (literally) bringing into question the disturbance of a social relationship whose effects are seen in the symbolic pattern of the logic of differences. The re-establishment of the disturbed relationship, like the re-establishment of physical balances, in itself entails the removal of the symptom and cure. In practice it is social (the confrontation of individuals or groups in question) or physical (the evolution of the symptom, the appearance of other illnesses) resistance which forces a reopening of the cycle "symptom-interpretation-re-establishment of the social relationship" until the moment when the peace of bodies and spirits allows it to be considered as closed.

But more often the diagnostic and therapeutic model is a virtual coherence model which opens the possibility, exclusive, alternative or simultaneous of two ways, one emphasising determination by cause, the other analysis by symptom. The examples in Togo that we have just presented correspond to one and the other of these procedures, but it is easy to see that they refer to the same principle of coherence.

Etiological interpretation, such as is operated in the system of shrines, immediately involves the consultation of the Fa oracle, who identifies the God (sometimes ancestor) causing the pain. But from the identification of the God flows that of the herbs likely to cure the illness of the young girl

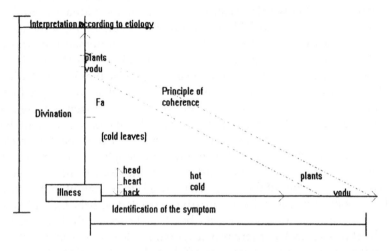

Interpretation according to the symptom

Diagnostic and therapeutic virtual coherence model

or woman chosen and called to initiate herself into the service of the God. A particular *vodu* is associated with particular plants which stem, as one has seen above, from his composition and constitute, in some fashion, his energy charge. The *vodu*-herbs relation introduces us to the universe where the coherence of the logic of differences is ordered, to which one has access through another entrance with the interpretation of the symptom. This symptom which is analysed in relation to a knowledge of the body and its balances which we have mentioned above, in itself entails treatment by herbs (warm or cold) but these herbs are themselves the property of a particular *vodu* to whom one must make a sacrifice for the treatment to take effect. In the first case the *vodu* is at the same time the cause and the remedy, in the second he is not associated with the curing of a pain for which he is not necessarily considered responsible. A few considerations however invite one to once more adjust the distinction between these two therapeutic procedures which anyway relates their common reference to a single principle of coherence. It often happens that the *bokonō* undertake to confirm through Fa the choice of plants made in regard of a single symptom. He then at the same time "announces" (it is the meaning of the term *bo*) the prescribed remedy and the name of the *vodu* concerned. Treatment by cause and treatment by symptom are, in fact, no longer distinguished than by a slight time difference in recourse to the oracle. The two procedures can even take place at the same time. This is the case when a serious illness is identified as personal, in other words as caused either by an individual's *legba* (his personal God with a two-fold effect, sometimes beneficent, sometimes maleficent), or by a disturbance whose cause is not named but whose remedy the Fa oracle can identify by addressing himself to *Mawu*. *Mawu* occupies a special place in the pantheon transmitted to the Guin and Mina by the Fon. He is a "superior" God in as much as that anything which cannot be imputed to another God, and by the same token recognized and named, can be attributed to him or treated by reference to him. In the case of a serious illness not claimed by another God, from what the oracle can uncover, *Mawu* is presented as the one who enlightens the divines on the nature of the remedies to administer to cure the sickness, not, properly speaking, as the cause of the latter. The cause is to be sought on the side of the personal divinities which tend to be associated with the individual's own body (since, as we have seen, the head, the heart and the back can be the object of sacrifice) or, more broadly, on the side of a personal destiny which it is more a matter of warding off than elucidating, since it is given once and for all, and in this sense is irrefutable, but which only has effect in certain circumstances.

Actually, consultation of the Fa oracle by an individual, in itself, corresponds to placing two figures in relation to each other. Any individual has his own signs the equivalent of our zodiac sign. Le Herissé has described how among the Fon, the adolescent concerned to know his personal symbol proceeded himself, assisted by the divines (*bokonō*), to the ritual elucidation of this sign, obtained by the random manipulation of nuts resulting in even and uneven combinations. It is only in "coming across" this personal configuration, revealed once and for all time, and which of course can be considered in itself as more or less favourable, with configurations which he obtains by an analogous method on the occasion of a given event and a particular consultation, that the *bokonō* can formulate an interpretation and propose a remedy. In this case (which, let it be noted, does not correspond to an absolutely fatalistic or deterministic conception of individual destiny) the procedure, which is simultaneously diagnostic and therapeutic, no longer distinguishes between the elucidation of the symptom and the identification of the cause.

In sum, the three logics define a differential and multi-dimensional logic (involved in what we have elsewhere called ideo-logic). Let us add that this logic is in no way a closed entity. In many respects it is only an uncertain line of direction which orientates the possibly antagonistic efforts of individuals and of groups to make up for the event. However these gaps and insufficiencies are not a factor ot plasticity. It is not itself the object of research and revision. Through it the unknown is always brought back to the possible and probable, to a more or less unstable compromise between the social norm and the reality of events. It must be added, concerning Africa or other continents subjected to more or less sudden and brutal forms of colonisation, that the degree of openness to the world and the exterior events of their ideological structure cannot in justice be estimated only in the light of these violent traumatisms and historical eruptions. When the measure of the adaptability of the system can be taken in better conditions (this qualification always remaining relative), it is revealed as larger than one would have been tempted to imagine. On the socio-political level, the adaptation of the coastal societies of West Africa to the mercantile demands of Europe in the 18th and 19th centuries bears witness to the flexibility of the lineal system.[31] One has just seen how the *vodu* in Togo attack the invasion of white religions without recourse to syncretism. It is certainly wrong to some extent to present as irrevocably closed, systems whose capacity for openness, on the contrary, some historical data allows us to perceive. Jack Goody[32] is well founded in criticising the too classic analysis of Horton.

However, the "Togolese" solution to the problem posed by the diffusion of the diverse avatars of Christian predication and of Western ideology is neither definitive nor widespread. The example of the prophet-healers of the Ivory Coast bears witness, for its part, at the same time to the impregnation of the persecutive pattern, linked to what we have proposed calling here the logic of references to and restatements of the notion of person which are inherent in it and correspond incontestably to a perversion of the earlier system. For prophets like Atcho in Ebrie country, Odjo in Adyoukrou country for example, the illness to be cured must certainly first be interpreted in term of social etiology, but the identification of the cause does not of itself entail cure. He who wishes to be cured must before everything purify himself first of all by confession. The settling of quarrels, the re-establishment of normal social relations is certainly desirable but, if they are not obtained, it is at least important, that it is not due to the deed of the patient. As, even in the perspective of non-Christian interpretation, any of the victim's errors eases the task of his aggressor, it is an easy step which, inverting the persecutive pattern, makes any victim a potential guilty party. In placing the responsibility for healing on the patient, the prophets tend to make any illness the expression of a fault, in the Christian sense of the term. Without giving up the therapeutic arsenal of traditional medicine, nor even the procedures of explanation and enquiry which, more or less, serve as substitutes for ordeal, the prophets intend to inculcate the meaning of pain into their patients. It is also a fact that pain has changed meaning from the moment when it no longer stemmed from the overall coherence of the logic of difference because this is less well known and, moreover, in new situations and for getting on with life (school, office, job, career), less meaningful. The new system corresponds to a principle of coherence so much more closed that one can see substituted for a symbolic framework of difference having reference to different social settings, an obsession with truth and prayer which leave patient and healer alone facing each other. As only the evolution of the symptom essentially matters, it is not surprising that there is, besides distraught or sceptical patients (always on the look-out for another way) and converted convalescents, prophets in turn worried and triumphal, each claiming for their part, the unique character of their calling, without being able to ignore that all around them places of prayer and salvation are multiplying.

****

Overall, the analysis of the ideo-logic conceived as the sum of the possible and the thinkable in a given society ought to permit the avoidance of two types of error whose nature the example of illness well illustrates. To ignore one of the three dimensions of the logic of illness leads one to play the endless game of explanation of symbolism, to abandon oneself to the fascination of the reciprocal cross-reference of the symbolically signifying to the socially signified which only ceases at the moment when the symbol no longer refers to anything but itself. The error is more precisely then to ignore that the individual can only understand the most intimate realities of his biological existence in terms which are always already social, but from his place within it — a place which is simultaneously assigned to him by an intellectual system, an institutional system which participated in it and individuals who occupy, by virtue of the same logic, another place within the system. Trying to define the logic of a system does not consist of denying its unequal structure and its means of perpetuation.

As for the possibilities of the system's change or evolution, which we have just suggested are certainly not nil, they seem very limited on the strict level of medical knowledge. Let us be clear about this point: the question can arise of knowing to what extent prolonged, systematic observations are not at the origin of the conceptions that certain societies make of heredity, of resemblance, of the relations of psychic forces between individuals, not to mention of their knowledge of the body and the action exercised by certain vegetal substances. In this sense any knowledge, even partial or theoretical, proceeds from experience. But the overall system to which this possibly experimentally produced knowledge is integrated responds much more to a requirement of meaning than a requirement of knowledge. Any meticulous knowledge is captured by the network of symbolic relations distributed over a universe which, as Levi-Strauss has shown, must have meaning for man before being able to be known: a requirement of significance in its principle, which the universe (in other words the man/nature relation so that man can perceive it) transforms into a signifying principle from the moment that the totality of symbolic relations, which are supposed to account for it but who, much rather, identify with it, come together in a logical whole. From then, any operation of knowledge, far from bearing upon this universe itself, refers to it as to the principle of coherence, which is the condition of all meaning.

One can admit, from this viewpoint, that any scientific progress passes through a metaphysical revolution (the one, perhaps, which consists of cutting man from nature before re-integrating him there), but the mistake consists in believing that the seeds of this revolution are present in certain "systems of thought" and not in others. The mistake, then, consists in distinguishing ethnocentrically that which concerns nature or empiricism and that which concerns personalisation or magic; in cutting off the logic of references from the logic of differences; in wrongly reducing, on the conceptual level, any social dimension to a causal dimension, and in constructing a diffusionist pattern which, come what may, accounts for the incessant refutation which sociological reality brings to these theoretical presuppositions. Certain American researchers have pushed this exercise of intellectual acrobatics far by enquiring, like George M. Foster[33] and Michael H. Logan,[34] into the relation between Spanish medicine and Amerindian medicine in Latin America. In both cases one first of all (briefly) recalls the history of the medicine of humours, more particularly the aspect which it assumed in America: the theory of hot and cold. One retraces its journey from Vedic India and ancient China to the Greeks, the Arabs and to Spain. Then one enquires into the coincidence of this theory with attested models in Latin America in the field of food, medical diagnosis and therapy. It is suggested that it stems from contact and diffusion first of all in "learned" circles, (1580, the creation of the chair in medicine at the University of Mexico; 1638, the creation the University of San Marco in Peru), then in "popular" circles, without being able to say anything precise about the modalities of this diffusion from one circle to another. The combination of hard categories (learned medicine, popular medicine) and of a soft sociology thus recreated a properly phantasmal history, anchored in the conviction that these authors have of the inequality of cultures and the benefits of what ethnology modestly calls diffusion.

This outrageous diffusionism stems from what must really be called a primitive anti-structuralism. To convince oneself it is enough to observe the artificial character of the arguments developed by our authors to cut the grass from under the feet of possible objectors. Certainly, admits Logan, one finds binary oppositions in Amerindian cosmologies and medicine, and Redfield demonstrated in 1941, that the systematic opposition of hot and cold was prior to European contact. But, he replies, the Spanish chroniclers, from where Redfield draws his information, perhaps projected their own conceptions onto the Indian ones: America, the Spanish inn in fact. Certainly Foster observes that the Spanish were impressed by the Indian healers and this observation well might press him to inquire into the direction of possible diffusion, there being nothing which would lead one to think that European medicine of the 16th and 17th centuries seemed, in the eyes of dazzled Indians, like a model of effectiveness. But quite the contrary, taking as read the fact of Spanish-American medical diffusion on the learned level, Foster can only consider oppositions of the hot/cold or dry/wet type evidenced in local Indian systems, as effects of this diffusion on the one part and of a transmission, proper to America, from the learned level to the popular level on the other part. The paradox reaches its height when Foster thinks he must nevertheless observe with certain specialists in Spanish folklore, that oppositions of this type did not exist in Spain at the "popular" level. One might expect that the discovery of such profound differences in the transmission of conceptual models would excite the interest of the anthropologist and the specialist. But apparently, on this point, Foster cares no more to change the hypothesis than to resolve the problems which it raises. This point of arrival from which nothing departs again signifies an impasse.

One wishes the diffusionists good luck when they tackle the African cosmological and sociological models. And one will conclude with two remarks. So-called "religious" anthropology proceeds in the way that so-called "religious" anthropology sometimes does when it more or less explicitly attempts to give an intellectual consistency to the notion of magic and assign it historical limits and geographic or ethnographic territories. The reduction of magic operated in all these procedures through the medium of a theory of social etiology of which only traces and survivals can be found with us in the West. This viewpoint, independent of the errors which it introduces, is decidedly non-anthropological. We wanted to suggest here that, if there was an anthropological and therefore social dimension of illness and, more broadly, elemental forms of event, it cannot be reduced to the definition of causes and is not the prerogative of certain societies.

Scientific analysis, a social relationship or a particular modality of relationship to the social, can also be considered as a cause of illness. But evidently the social/illness relationship cannot be reduced to a causal link. Notions of work and production perhaps constitute the intermediary categories between illness and society which permit one to think of them in a coherent way in relation to each other. Without doubt one can and must distinguish in this type of relationship between purely causal relations (professional illness) and relations less and less identifiable to an exclusively causal link (from so-called psycho-somatic illness to cardio-vascular illness, from illness in general to regimes supposed to prevent them, from regimes with images of the individual and the person, about which one no longer knows if they control them or are controlled by them). One would abandon to the specialists the legitimate and stimulating task of drawing up the individual, ecological, sociological and exterior (viruses for example) factors which are the origin of certain illnesses (one thinks here notably of the work of J. Ruffie on the origin of certain cancers which in fact demand recourse to comparative ethnography). But to the reconstitution one would primarily attach more or less share ideas, images more or less received by everybody (this "more or less" depends on differences of cultural capital and situation within the system, which are perhaps not decisive in this respect) and whose grounding medical authority reinforces since it denounces scourges, types of consumption (fats, alcohol, tobacco, drugs) which one cannot relate to some lifestyles and beyond that, some relationships of productions including those on the international scale. Illness would not be alone in this. It is certain for example that the notion of accident (with its institutional corollaries: insurance, prevention) also comes into the elaboration of a referential universe whose composition and attributes can appear as if of a religious nature where they point to and impose, before all else and like all religions, a certain idea of Man. The religion of Westerners, the one to which they all belong, is perhaps essentially the totality of representations which systematise their daily practice and whose architecture and coherence, the anthropologist, attentive to their emotions, their imprudences, their regimes and their excesses, will perhaps one day be able to glimpse — having, on this occasion, taken a path opposite to the one imposed on him by Africa, America or Oceania, whose systems he believed he knew and whose individuals he did not dare imagine.

NOTES

1. C. Castoriadis *L'institution imaginaire de la société*, Paris, Le Seuil, 1975.
2. R. Establet, "Culture et ideológie", Cahiers marxistes-leninistes, no. 12–13, June–Oct. 1966, pp. 15–18.
3. Luc de Heusch, *Pourquoi l'épouser? et autres essais*, Paris, Gallimard, 1971.
4. Henry E. Sigerist, *A History of Medicine*, vol. 1, Primitive and Archaic Medicine, Oxford University Press, 1951.
5. Placide Tempels, *La philosophie bantoue*, Paris, Présence africaine, 1949.
6. George M. Foster, "Disease etiologies in non-Western medical systems" *American Anthropologist*, **LXXVIII**, 1976, pp. 773–782.
7. George P. Murdock, S.F. Wilson and V. Frederick, "World distribution of theories of illness", *Ethnology*, **XVII**, 1978, pp. 449–470. Also found in: G.P. Murdock, Theories of Illness: a World Survey, Pittsburgh, University of Pittsburgh Press, 1980.
8. Maria M. Suarez, "Etiology, hunger and folk diseases in the Andes", *Journal of Anthropological Research*, **XXX**, 1974, pp. 41–54.
9. Reo F. Fortune, *Sorcerers of Dobu: the Social Anthropology of the Dobu Islanders* of the Western Pacific, London, G. Routledge, 1932. French translation: *Sorciers de Dobu*, Paris, Maspero, "Bibliothique d'anthropologie", 1972.
10. J. Middleton and E.H. Winter, eds., *Witchcraft and Sorcery in East Africa*, London, Routledge & Kegan Paul, 1963.
11. B. Malinowski, *The Dynamics of Culture Change, an Inquiry into Race Relations in Africa*, Oxford University Press, 1945. French translation: *Les dynamiques de l'evolution culturelle*, Paris, Payot, "Bibliotheque scientifique", 1970.
12. Max Gluckman, *Order and Rebellion in Tribal Africa: Collected Essays*, London, Cohen and West, 1963.
13. Eva Gillies, "Causal criteria in African classifications of disease", in J.B. Loudon, ed., *Social Anthropology and Medicine*, London, Academic Press, 1976, pp. 358–395.
14. Victor W. Turner, *The Drums of Affliction*, Oxford, Clarendon Press, 1986. French translation: *Les tambours d'affliction*, Paris, Galimard, 1972.
15. E. H. Ackerknecht, "Natural diseases and rational treatment in primitive medicine", *Bulletin of the History of the Medicine*, **XIX**, 1946, pp. 467–497. Reprinted under the title "Naturalistic and supernaturalistic diagnosis and treatments" in *Medicine and Ethnology: Selected Essays*, Baltimore, John Hopkins Press, 1971, pp. 135–161.
16. H. A. Junod, *The Life of a South African Tribe*, 2nd ed., vol., London, 1927.
17. Karl G. Lindbom, *The Akamba in British East Africa*, 2nd ed., Uppsala, 1920.

18. G. W. Harley, *Native African Medicine, with Special Reference to its Practice in the Mano Tribe of Liberia*, Cambridge, Mass., Harvard University Press, 1941.

19. E. H. Ackerknecht, "Primitive Medicine", in *Transactions of the New York Academy of Science*, ser. II, VIII, 1947, pp. 26–37. Reprinted under the title "Typical aspects" in *Medicine and Ethnology*, op. cit., pp. 17–29.

20. Evans-Pritchard remarks that in 1965 (in *Theories of Primitive Religion*), as Jean Pouillon usefully reminds us in his "Comments on the verb to believe" (in *The Symbolic Function*, a work cited below), and Durkheim already did in *The Elemental Forms of Religious Life*, noting that "primitive people" do not feel they are dealing with "irrational" forces when they carry out fertility rites.

21. Michel Foucault, *Histoire de la folie à l'âge classique*, new edition, Paris, Gallimard, 1972 (1st. ed. 1961).

22. Robin Horton, "African traditional thought and Western science", *Africa*, XXXVII, 1967, pp. 50–71, 155–187.

23. Françoise Héritier, "Fécondité et stérilité: la traduction de ces notions dans le champ idéologique au stade préscientifique", in Evelyne Sullerot, ed., *Le fait féminin*, Paris, Fayard, 1978, pp. 289–306.

24 Françoise Héritier, "Symbolique de l'inceste et de sa prohibition", in *La fonction symbolique: essais d'anthropologie*, collected by M. Izard and P. Smith, Paris, Gallimard, 1979, pp. 209–243.

25. Marc Augé, *Pouvoirs de vie, pouvoirs de mort*, Paris, Flammarion, 1977.

26. R. Pazzi, *L'homme eve, aja, gèn, fon- et son univers*, Lome, 1976 (a document with many contributors).

27. Pierre Verger, *Notes sur le culte des Orisa et Vodun à Bahia, au Brésil et à l'ancienne côte des Esclaves en Afrique*, Dakar, French Institute of Black Africa, 1957.

28. Richard F. Burton, *A Mission to Gelele, King of Dahomey*, edited with an introduction and notes by C. W. Newbury, London, Routledge & Kegan Paul, 1966 (1st. ed. 1864).

29. A. Le Hérissé, *L'ancien royaume du Dahomey*, Paris, 1911.

30. Melville J. Herskovits, *Dahomey, an Ancient West African Kingdom*. 2 vol., New York, 1938.

31. M. Augé, "L'organisation du commerce précolonial en Basse Côte d'Ivoire et ses effets sur l'organisation sociale des populations côtières", in Cl. Meillassoux, ed., *L'évolution du commerce en Afrique de l'Quest*, London, Oxford University Press, for the International African Institute, 1971, pp. 153–167.

32. J. Goody, *La raison graphique*, Paris, Editions de Minuit, 1979 (translation of: *The Domestication of the Savage Mind*, Cambridge, 1977).

33. G. M. Foster, "Relationships between Spanish and Spanish-American folk medicine", *Journal of American Folklore*, LXVI, no. 261. New York, John Wiley, 1978.

34. M. H. Logan, "Anthropological research on the hot-cold theory of disease: some methodological suggestions", *Medical Anthropology*, I, no. 4, 1977. pp. 87–112.

Chapter 2

THE NEED FOR MEANING: THE EXPLANATION OF ILL FORTUNE AMONG THE SENUFO

N. Sindzingre

In Western societies as well as in the so-called traditional societies, if there is one pursuit of meaning that particularly affects all individuals, it is the quest for the origin of biophysiological disorder of illness. The reminder of the existence of organs and the sudden noise they produce are, to paraphrase Lerich's definition of health, raw and universal body information. A merely phenomenological occurrence at first, illness is that impenetrable and strictly personal event which, starting from a certain threshold established by society, converts the state of health, perhaps equivalent to "normality", "productivity" and social integration, into another state: the state of illness. Like the "phase transitions" in the physical world (e.g. a liquid becoming a jelly) illness involves, for the individual but also for his social group, a binary change of state and can be regarded, as it was by M. Augé, as the image *par excellence* of the event. Indeed, if the organism is considered as a whole that functions in certain conditions, then illness, whether it is conceived as an entity or as a disorder or imbalance, is the paradigm of what can happen to or, in spinozistic terms, what affects a body.

In any "conception of the world" an event requires, by definition, an explanation. It has its place in a process of causality, where it represents a cause, *a fortiori* illness. Since illness is characterized by a decrease in an individual's capacities, all societies have endeavoured not only to find a cause, but also to eradicate this event. His very aims and methods place the anthropologist in a privileged position to know that everywhere, illness immediately gives rise to a host of questions. Why? Why me? Why now? How did it happen to me? Who or what is at the origin of the misfortune that has stricken me? The question of causality, the subject-matter of this study, is therefore inseparable from the actual realization that there is a physiological problem, and there are two reasons for this. On the one hand, it is part of the empirical and omnipresent reality which it is the anthropologist's task to observe. This is especially true in traditional societies, since it is precisely there that the forms of pathology, which concern the majority of the population, are least under control, and there that they are also always related to an explanatory system with a more or less structured and perceptible code.

On the other hand, it is a fact of principle that illness and causal representations are inseparable, inasmuch as illness is, as we have seen, the preeminent event and individual affect. This is why, as regards causality in an analysis of the representations and practices of a given society, it is so often difficult to distinguish between the categories of illness and those of misfortune in general. In other words, as far as explanations are concerned, they are homologous. Each characterizes a change of state, a shift away from the normal state of things. Both sets of categories are regarded as *effects*, and thus as stages of an interpretation, even if, from other angles such as the semantic and obviously the pragmatic, these categories may be clearly distinguishable.

I. ANTHROPOLOGICAL CAUSALITY

After these introductory remarks, it must be remembered that anthropology has a long analytic tradition in the field of illness. As part of this tradition, the argument developed here endeavours to evaluate the notion of causality, of ill-fortune, and of biophysical disorder in traditional, mainly African societies where Western models and facilities are not dominant, using data from one particular society, the Fodonon, a Senufo sub-group of the Ivory Coast. Moreover, the possible ways to remedy the disorder, intended to "restore the balance", will be dealt with in their relation to causal thinking. We thus hope to show certain specific features of the explanatory models of "illness" in non-Western societies, as against societies where the biomedical scientific discourse or the discourse of the "great" universalist religions, such as Christianity or Islam, prevail. We are speaking here of predominant models, because it is clear that in the regions concerned the models are closely interconnected.

Compared to other theories on the interpretation of illness, philosophical, historical or biomedical theories for example, the anthropological theory is different because of the innate specificity of its approach. It regards illness as a representation and therefore as a social fact; it considers illness as an intellectual *and* pragmatic production, "representation" does not refer only to thoughts or words, but also to behaviour, the production of a given group, as a particular division in a social reality. By hypothesis the approach is "holistic". It is true that for a long time ill-fortune and illness were not studied independently. Very often they were integrated in global analyses of thinking and of "religious", "magical", and "ritual" practices, beginning in the days of Durkheim and Mauss, or of symbolic systems, for instance, in Evans-Pritchard's studies on magic and witchcraft among the Azande, Levi-Strauss's work on the rules classifying primitive thought, or V. Turner's study of Ndembu atonement for "affliction" rituals.[1]

The dependency of the field of illness, and its treatment as a specific facet of religious thinking, an aspect of the use of symbolic categories or rites, is due precisely to the fact that members of traditional communities immediately put forward causality, and to the treatments of illness used locally. All illness or ill-fortune requires an interpretation and that interpretation reflects the social relations and representations typical of a society. Evans-Pritchard's famous example of a tile falling off the roof of an Azande barn and hitting someone will inevitably give rise to the following questions: The tile could have fallen earlier, or later, or not at all, so why did it fall just then? Why did it hit me, or him? The victim asks himself these questions and so do those who, by virtue of their social relationships with him, are in a position to ask them. Being the object of ill-fortune is fundamentally unjust to anyone, and it implies a need to find a meaning and to insert it into a chain of cause and effect. In other words, it implies a need to find an explanation. An explanation is especially warranted in the event of death, even if the victim is by definition no longer there to hear it. In the Azande community, sorcery, which is the gift of certain lineage members and the idiom of inter-and intra-lineage relationships, provides a dominant model of the causality of ill-fortune. In other communities, the models hinge on other representations. They lay greater stress on the "vertical" dimension by including instances such as ancestors, or are based on powers which animate both space and filiation groups, the "spirits", or on a person's actions, such as taboo transgressions.

A common feature of these various approaches to the interpretation is, briefly speaking, the exogenous nature of causality: the situation which triggers off the trouble is the result of factors outside the victim of the ill-fortune which can be human or non-human; visible or invisible; subjectivized and endowed with intentionality or impersonal; sorcerers, spirits, "fetishes", ancestors. It can also result from an inherent social rule, such as the taboos related to certain circumstances, objects or people. These factors as a whole, "distant" causes in a way, are an answer to the question "why?", while other intermediary determinism of the world of physical empirical regularities, for example, may specifically indicate the process in all societies, catching a cold, burning oneself, etc. There is no such thing as a society evolving in pure speculation; they all possess a different knowledge drawn from the observation of these regularities ("common sense").

The state of illness, then, sets in motion a process of withdrawal of the victim's responsibility ("exculpation") as has been shown by Parsons (and Gluckman for anthropology[2]); in this his ill-fortune does not depend on his will. This is also true of our societies, though in traditional societies the contents clearly differ, for example, from the chemical, biological, and psychological contents that were introduced by biomedical knowledge. Biomedical science clearly separates illness from ill-fortune and links illness to physiological processes devoid of all intentionality or immanence, basic qualities of the categories used in a scientific approach. Moreover, attributing the cause to an outside element is not the same as fully excusing the victim, nor does this mean that he was passive in the causal development. He can be at the origin of the onset of illness, or of the activity of exogenous instances, for example by adopting an attitude which does not comply with the social norms. Often the victim of a sorcery attack may already stand out because of characteristics, features or behaviour which is socially reprehensible. For example, they may be excessive ("too much" good luck, or "too much" bad luck, etc.) The transgressor of a taboo who is penalized by an illness could have been more careful and there are occasions where to a certain extent he knowingly committed the transgression. However, this does not call into question the possible presence of other connecting elements in the causality which are foreign to the subject. Hence the variations in feelings of guilt, in the sense that a person is the cause of his own misfortune, depending on the society or vicissitudes of history. Studies of the kinds of treatments which the Ivory Coast "prophet" A. Atcho administers illustrate this by giving a plausible explanation of causality in terms of "paranoia".[3]

What matters here is that the exogenous characteristic of the factors explaining illness, be they sorcerers or powers from the village universe or from the bush (or even harsh working conditions or inextricable family situations) necessarily implies that the explanation makes real sense only in reference to a given religious, symbolic and social organization. An explanatory statement always has a social referent; an irregular, pathological situation is only experienced and treated as such because it is an integral part of a whole. This is why recent developments in so-called medical anthropology or in ethnomedicine, mainly in English-speaking countries, by isolating the facts of the illness to present them as postulates of an independent anthropological object, sometimes also empty them of their substance and deprive them of any meaning. They are disconnected from their pragmatic context and from social causality. Sometimes they even evoke economic Robinsonades. However, the attempt is licit and may well have followed the example of political or economic anthropology. It is of great interest to circumscribe the distinctive features of the field of illness in relation to other ritual and symbolic representations and institutions. On the borderline of sorcery, religious cults of possession or divination, the field of ill-fortune and of illness is nevertheless not a priori limited to them. It would, therefore, be wrong to consider these as homologous phenomena. Some remarkable contributions from G. Lewis, J.B. Loudon and A. Young[4] have illustrated this specificity.

Nevertheless, the hypothesis that the facts of illness may have a meaning in themselves which would open the way for comparative studies of the "cross-cultural" type clashes with the aporias engendered by the premises of medical anthropology. Schematically, these can be divided into two categories. First of all, it is postulated that illness is a subject that groups a series of social facts, nosologies, diagnostic methods, therapeutic institutions and modalities, whose inner workings call for analysis with the help of concepts constructed for this purpose, such as "medical pluralism" (A. Kleinman)[5] as a plurality of therapeutic possibilities within one and the same society, which is not very fruitful, or psychosociological concepts, such as the "social construction of reality" (P.L. Berger and T. Luckmann), of restricted anthropological scope. The debate on social causality plays only a minor role here alongside other variables. Sometimes the result is a shift of the analysis leading to an essentially descriptive approach (for example, the study of nosological categories in a given society), a sociological approach (the study of therapeutic institutions available in a given area), or even a medicalized approach (the study of the expression of a given syndrome within a given group). These are all legitimate approaches, but do not belong to anthropology *strictu sensu*, which takes a qualitative standpoint, offering both an overall and a microscopic view.

Perhaps the problem of causality under consideration falls back on the notion of an aetiology typical of "non-Western medical systems", where the Western medical model is still used as the yardstick. Apart from the limitations intrinsic to this reduction, such an approach cannot but produce descriptive and typological schema that are too general to be useful. Thus, following L.B. Glick, G.M. Foster[6] also admits that "the most important fact concerning illness" is recognizing not so much the pathological process as the "underlying cause", because according to him, we shall conclude further on that this is not always the case, most diagnoses and treatments are arrived at by detecting causal factors. It is an attempt to propose a possibly universal distinction between "person-alistic aetiologies", involving agents with their own volition, and "natu-ralistic aetiologies", involving forces of nature (cold, etc.). Besides the fact that this division does not take into account the typical features of each society (and in this aspect the widest variations are possible), it creates more problems than it solves, and among them the extremely complex problem of the explanatory value, of the *raison d'être* of world theories based on "personal" entities, and of differences between them and the scientific theories or the "great" religions.

In general, because of its own premises, medical anthropology cannot easily escape the influence of the "paradigm" of Western medicine, to quote T. Kuhn,[7] and its concomitant objectives and theories; underlying criteria of effectiveness, selection of variables considered as "medical" in the biomedical system (symptoms, healers, techniques, etc.). On the one hand, the mechanisms of symbolic effectiveness are unknown here and, on the other hand, as A. Young[8] points out, the Western "paradigm" cannot explain the existence of beliefs and practices which are ineffective according to biomedical criteria, but are otherwise perfectly effective, i.e., appropriate to the cognitive and predictive universe of the societies considered. Nor can it explain the reason for their survival in societies where recourse may be had to the Western model with its objective therapeutic power in the form of hospitals and dispensaries. Perhaps only an epistemological reflexion on the different kinds of knowledge involved here can shed light on the points of similarity and dissimilarity. The scientific paradigm cannot a priori claim to assess all cases of systems set up outside it.

Another presupposition of the ethnomedical approach, linked to the previous one, involves the very notion of "system". Whereas it is quite acceptable to isolate a medical system in our societies, medical sociology does so, the data from traditional societies where the borderline between the field of illness and other related fields, religion and rites in particular, is virtually unnoticeable or covers the social tissue as a whole, preclude the use of the biomedical systemic model as a referent for analysis. Neither the nosologies, i.e., identifying and naming the disorders, nor the causality schemas, nor the therapeutic institutions a priori form a system. Likewise, the studies focusing on local taxonomies and classifications referring to biomedical parameters (organic symptoms, types of illnesses, for instance) may well omit certain categories and connections. Troubles affecting a group, for example, the series of infant deaths among the Senufo which make a lineage feel "ill", and which in this case was related to a sexual transgression by a woman of the matrilineage, or disorders with no apparent organic foundation, etc. They also avoid the problem of the social decision by which an individual or a group feels and is considered to be ill, and that of the decision labelling the illness. The terms used to designate an illness may vary over time. The choices are made according to "extra-medical" criteria, collective strategies, for example.

If the observer were able to extract a series of classifiable date, causes or symptoms, they would often prove impossible to organize into hierarchical and comprehensive taxonomies, but would rather follow a different type of logic, of the paradox, or of the "disjunctive synthesis" (either... or...) type. As the Senufo example illustrates, the final concrete allocation (such and such a symptom, such and such a cause) results from a practical decision and may fluctuate depending on the peculiarities of life histories, social tensions, individual and collective interests and strategies. According to J. Goody,[9] we can also add that the form of the taxonomy, like a painting implying simultaneity and totalisation, involves patterns of thought unknown to unlettered societies.

II. EXPLAINING ILLNESS: THE SENUFO EXPERIENCE

What characterizes the processes of explaining and dissipating ill-fortune in traditional societies? We shall endeavour to answer that question with material collected among the Fodonon, a Senufo community of the Ivory Coast. Our conclusions are certainly not applicable to other societies, precisely because they are coextensive with a particular social organization and because the system of symbolic representations on which they are based is, by definition, unique. They differ, for instance, from the Bantu societies and from the interpretations and therapies of the *nganga* "healers", which at the same time make a diagnosis, assess the causes and provide a remedy, in a way which is more evocative for the Western observer.

However, certain features, in particular the full implicitness of exogenous variables, the importance of agent-elements of the local conception of the physical universe, spirits and powers, and of the human universe, ancestors, are largely recurrent in African societies at least. They are recurrent in causal shape and content, in internal functioning and in the categories used. Drawing from the fields traditionally called "religious" or "magic", they lead us to reconsider this type of division.

First, we shall describe the representations and the explanation schema, or the possible causal connections, as well as their independence from the process of resolution (possible practices and representations of the a priori causality). Secondly, we shall examine the logic behind the choice of a particular causality and therapy. The choice is here made by divination and the initial choice of a therapist (an exercise of a posteriori causality). Let us not forget that "representation" in this case does not mean a certain idea obtaining in a society, but in the Durkheimian sense, beliefs and judgments that are backed up by real practices. The data from the Senufo show that at least three degrees of coherence come into play. They schematically govern the designation and the causality of the troubles, their particular interpretation (divination) and the therapy. Their unity stems from practices extrinsic to the field of ill fortune in the strict sense that originate in the lineal social organization, typical of the Fodonon.

1. Possible A Priori Causality

This is the first register of coherence, the causal connections that each individual can make a priori between the trouble (ill-fortune or a physiological symptom) and its cause. Like any society, including our own, the Fodonon take an unfortunate event and establish a series of connections based on a set of representations ordering their daily life. It is not pertinent here to distinguish "popular" knowledge from scientific knowledge, to quote a frequently used distinction, because first of all the level of specialization is very low since everyone has access to this knowledge and also because the viewpoint taken here is based on an average kind of knowledge possessed by every person, before the real therapeutic itinerary starts. This journey will determine "afterwards" and "step by step" the actual type of beliefs and practices that are applicable in each case. If we start with the question: "What is said and what happens when the threshold of illness is reached?", the distinction between the two kinds of knowledge is of secondary importance, since it does not determine the causes or the therapeutic institutions.

The Fodonon are peasants. They live in village communities in a tightly-structured matrilineal society, forming a group which is not centralized by any political institution. The lineage culture is land-centred, as witnessed by the use of arable land and the organization in village districts. The community, which is made up of the separate districts surrounding the founding lineages, is governed by a council of district leaders headed by a "master of the land", a *primus inter pares*, who stands for the symbolic integrity of the land and is responsible for good relations between the people and the *madabele*, "spirits of the land", who are its original owners. In this society, where power is manifested mainly through a supplementary distribution of "authorities" in a particular area (land, district, lineage, cult, divination, remedies, etc.), the beliefs and institutions concerning ill-fortune take on an original dimension, since, unlike in state societies, they are as fully developed as other fields of village life (male initiation rituals, organization in districts or lineages). They are not secondary, but form specific spheres of activity utilized when necessary. The analysis of illness is thus a field which runs through the community as a whole. The community is also well structured by both ethnic and ritual practices emphasizing village unity and equality and also obedience to those rules, the many taboos in particular, which in this context contribute largely to the establishment and survival of the social order.

Before discussing the forms and content of the causality of illness and ill-fortune, we must remind the reader that these notions are part of the everyday and omnipresent round. In a real community based on social uniformity, misfortune and illness form unacceptable gaps and are essential events in individual existence which are necessarily part of an explanation. Whether he wants to or not, the observer is, as other studies of African societies prove, continually faced with questions on the cause of "bad luck" whatever its form: personal illness or illness in the family, sterility and no descendants, a series of deaths in the lineage or residence group and poor crops, to mention only the most frequent examples. As socio-economic changes reach the Fodonon, just as they do other African societies, the content changes gradually owing to new models of urbanization and economic inequality: frustrated aspirations to earn a wage, free choice of a spouse, "wealth".

First of all the contents of the categories of ill-fortune: the Fodonon distinguish illness/*yaama* as a physiological syndrome from those kinds of ill-fortune of which illness is a sub-section. The other categories are: *yewuo*/the "black figure" and *tete*/*toro* which bring bad luck and ill fortune, and are marked by a repetition of the events.

However, in a concrete situation these notions are not so different and the categorization of this kind of disorder in the end always depends on practical criteria. When ill-fortune recurs and piles up on an individual or one of his kin groups, the threshold of perception being variable by definition, it marks a new change of state, not only of the state of health (*tyeri nyime*/"freshness of the body") of the victim of the illness/*yaama*, but first of a predisposition. Repeated illness and ill-fortune are the signs of something else, the signs that their victim is the object of another sort of ill-fortune, the *tete* or *toro*. These labels in their turn provide an explanation, and in that sense they justify the person's further ill-fortune. From this point onwards it is because a person has *tete* that he is destined to suffer ill-fortune. Such a system where notions may interchange according to a collective evaluation foreign to them, reveals how vain it is to attempt to draw up taxonomies of medical categories with an uncertain outcome.

Furthermore, from the point of view of the causality's form, ill-fortune and illness are not severable either, since either one or the other may well be the effect of the same *finite series* of causes. Sorcery, for instance, can be a possible cause of a predisposition to an unfortunate destiny as well as of any organic symptom.

The study of the list of possible aetiologies and symptoms underlined features common to other African societies: one the one hand, the *finite number* of categories involved in the explanation of a disorder that can take the place of the cause, and, on the other, their coexistensiveness with the field traditionally called "religion": God, powers and spirits, etc. It may sound like a trivial observation, but it shows the difficulties that occur in the analysis when words have to be used that are burdened with a century of conceptual anthropological construction, but a different approach is not feasible. It also makes us wonder about the existence of attributes typical of "religion" and "medicine". The observation also illustrates the degree of openness of a field usually circumscribed by medical anthropology. We could even ask ourselves if there is a causal conception of ill-fortune that is not founded on a general conception of the physical world and based on a human and a non-human world, and which does not implicate, in variable forms, close, direct, instrumental and distant causes, instances qualifying the inobservables of the physical world, to use J. Skorupski's[10] expression or the religious "absolutely other". In a stimulating study R. Horton[11] insisted on the following idea: in traditional societies it would seem that when the "way of thinking" induces causal inferences meant to explain the world of experience, then recourse is had to entities of the "non-human agent" type which have the value here of theoretical and sometimes transcendental concepts. The notion of causality activated by these "religious" agents supplies a coherent connection between the empirical world with its regularities and its anomalies, and the non-observable, here the "theoretical hypothesis". It is above all a way of describing and explaining the world. According to Horton, it is prediction, explanation and control, all in one.

The Fodonon hold that "ill-fortune" and illness, which is a particularly acute form of ill-fortune, are connected in the domain of what is *possible*, i.e., outside a concrete collective or individual pathological situation, to a finite series of categories, instances and facts. Here causality stands for this connection in its most simple meaning: event A is said to be caused by B, its occurrence depends on B. The delicate question of the direction of the inference will be mentioned only because connections vary according to whether we start with the disorder or with its cause. This is consistent with the actual exercise of causality where the problem does not occur. These categories are listed in the following table. They englobe the entire field of possible causality for the Fodonon. The table is meant as a memory aid only, for it does not correspond to any empirical situation. It is possible to arrive at this series retrospectively, after compilation of many explanations and processes. This is why it is not a taxonomy. The causal categories are not manifest in a systematized whole, they are chosen according to practical circumstances, their connections to disorders vary and as the table will show, they do not belong to classification levels which are logically homogeneous. Among other things, they blend one into another and they share common features. So a twin can be a sort of ancestor, an ancestor a sort of fetish, the creator a sort of *yawige*, "thing that pursues", etc. Some, such as the *yawige* and the taboo can also be the attributes of other categories. Ethnological thought a priori presents itself as a paradox which disappears when extrinsic social choices

Senufo Causal Categories

	Senufo Terms	*Specifications*
A mechanical factor X		"natural" illnesses
God ("Illnesses of God")	Kulotyolo	illnesses without any other discernible cause
The "Guardian" spirit of the individual	Yirigeflo	
Twins of the matrilineage	Ngambele	
The ancestors of the matrilineage	Kubele	agents which fall or descend upon the individual
The fetishes of the matrilineage	Sandoho	
Spirits of places (Earth, the bush, rivers)	Mãdebele	
The sorcerers of the matrilineage	debele	illnesses "thrust upon" the individual
Magic objects and fetishes, individual or cultural	yasungo, katyene	
The "pursuit", the *nyuma* of animals killed in the brush or of corpses	Yawige	illnesses acquired by contamination
Transgression of rules	yafungo	Rules which the individual is bound to by lineage (objects, status, etc.)

are made. Nevertheless, the list of these categories is fixed and covers all the possible causes that now exist.[12]

The table shows that many explanations are possible for a given affliction. Before going into any details, we should point out that all these explanations, and this is where in their forms they resemble scientific causality, have both a predictive and a retrospective function. If an individual or group shows a symptom which is socially observed and named, then the cause or causes are among these categories. If a category comes into action, then certain unfortunate events of an endless list of possibilities that may or may not preferentially refer to the agent are very likely to occur. Such a model of causality is therefore dissymetric, since it links *infinite* events to *finite* entities, depending on the sense in which the explanation moves: explaining a past event that has already taken place or speculating and forecasting the future. One of my children falls ill. It is a real event that I can relate only to one or other of the possible causes that my society places at my disposal and that may refer to real event (my transgression of a taboo, for example) or to inobservable events (the malevolent action of a sorcerer).

Conversely, the person who, knowingly or not, transgresses a taboo or is in contact with powers that could cause an illness can only foresee that he will be the victim of any kind of ill-fortune, which, when it occurs, will be related to this cause or to another, through divination. So, the causality which is here illustrated connects the infinite domain of ill-fortune with that of finite causes, and from the point of view of real situations, explaining and foreseeing are two different things. The big problem of religious anthropology concerning the fallibility of traditional models emerges here. It is the problem of restricting the field of experience in models that do not leave scope for any alternative, even if outside representations are assimilated in such a traditional causal category, for instance, the *zar* spirits underlying possession in Ethiopia, some of which are of outside origin, or white origin, etc. It is this "circularity" of the first register of coherence, of the explanation, that we want to emphasize here.

The first causal category, which relates a disorder to a "mechanical" factor, a determinist causality in a way, points towards an aspect which is sometimes minimized in ethnological studies that emphasize models of mystic aggression (sorcery) or else overestimated in studies of an ethno-scientific nature. Like all societies, the Fodonon are perfectly capable of considering that a common cold, for example, can be caused by having caught a cold, without necessarily searching for other factors. We must also point out that this category does not fully cover all innocuous disorders, as could have been expected, because the explanation partially depends on the denomination made spontaneously by the patient himself or by an "elder" close to him. Some nosological entities that are very frequent and that have an uncertain outcome, such as "hot body" / *tyefuru*, do not automatically follow from this type of connection. They are the very example of illnesses that have multiple social aetiologies.

Let us add that the determinist, formal nature of a connection does not necessarily entail a rational conception of the world following the example of scientific thought. It already implies a symbolic selection (present in every society) of the relevant facts. Saying that contact of the skin with *bolongo* grain results in acute pruritus / *toho*, already implies choosing and symbolically connecting separate categories in the field of experience. Determinist connections specify a type of causality of which Evans-Pritchard noted the importance in relation to Azande explanation theories. They cannot be rightly identified with the laws that are established by scientific discourse, even if they look similar. Moreover, it is relevant neither for the Fodonon nor for the anthropologist to detect in them premises of a biomedical *ratio* in them.

God / *kulotyolo* may be said to cause ill-fortune, but ultimate cause of the world and of any event. This causal category is not homogenous with the others in the sense that in a conditional statement such as "if p..., then q" God cannot take the place of "p". So, "if kulotyolo..., then such and such an ailment will affect someone" is impossible. A "generalized cause", "a unique common element that participates in all causes", according to the felicitous expression of Evans-Pritchard,[13] then God is a causal "last resort" invoked only when no other is possible. It seems that this idea of an entity that does not intervene in the human world, an ultimate cause of everything, exists in a number of African societies, therefore prudence is called for when transposing religious categories deriving from revealed religions. As Horton would say, it is a necessary transcendental hypothesis englobing the other entities of the physical world (ancestors, spirits, ...) that could be distinguished depending on their relative proximity to the universe of human social reality.

The third possible causal category, the "guardian" spirit of the individual, has precisely that "closer" relation with humans. A component of the person, *virigefolo* / he who creates, who "brings out", is an entity that "precipitates", that initiates the coming into the world of the individual and then is born and dies with them. It is forced to remain protector to the individual it has created but can also be easily offended laying down a series of prescriptions and taboos (often concerning food, sometimes sex), such as wearing the insignia, etc. The paradoxical character of causality lies here in the modalities of its advent. Each person knows that he has a *virigefolo*; in everyone's life the process evolves as follows: during adolescence one falls ill; a diviner, a major factor of effective interpretation, is consulted and he assigns the cause of the illness to the "creator". This is how *virigefolo* manifests itself to its protégé and specifies the particular obligations that it demands in return for its benevolence which may vary according to the individual. Subsequent failure to respect these demands may lead to ill-fortune and illness for the "host" individual, which is generally related to food. Inversely, many disorders ("stomach-ache", scabies) are related by divination and sometimes by "spontaneous" interpretation to a transgression of these taboos or a negligence of these prescriptions (especially sacrificial). The individual may have committed the transgression knowingly, which happens when a person who, feeling that he has a surfeit of taboos, finds that respecting them provides little protection against ill-fortune. He may also have been unaware of his transgression, for example, because he did not know which ingredients were used to prepare a meal that he ate. Here then we have the *retrospective* conception of the explanation which is moreover irrefutable, a fragment of the conception which we have already mentioned and which is founded on circular reasoning. An instance of ill-fortune, an illness, is one day interpreted as an indication of *virigefolo*, which then commands respect under the threat of identical ills during the person's whole life. This entity owes its very existence to ill-fortune. It is *strictu sensu* a possible theory of it through the notion of taboo and of its transgression, an authentic "operator" of a large part of the explanation of illness. An instance that also explains good luck retrospectively (the taboos and prescriptions have been respected), it is a transcendent form of the hazards of individual life. The foundation of the belief is thus not challenged, that would introduce a conception other than causes and effects, a "way out" avoiding this connection. Ill-fortune will always occur in the life of everyone who, corroborating the initial infringement, will prove the existence of *virigefolo* and the rightfulness of its demands.

A similar causality schema lies at the basis of the fourth possible causal category: the twins of the matrilineage, *ngambele*, power of the Fodonon universe, like God and the individual creator. Every matrilineage has certain "cointensive" powers which are guarantors of its existence and its durability: ancestors/*kubele*, spirits/*madebele*, fetishes/*vasungyi*, *sandoho* and twins are all conceived as potential causes of the events that affect the life of every member of the matrilineage. The Fodonon, a society where the representations highly value the matrilineage as a community of the living and the dead in continuity and in depth, prove to what extent the explanation of ill-fortune relies on their own social structures. Five of the causal categories, if we include intra-lineal sorcery (witchcraft), are powers existing in every matrilineage. The causality of the event here largely stems from beliefs regarding the theory of filiation. This feature, with its specific form and content, can be found in most African societies. Once the twins actually appear in a matrilineage, they remain there forever as a power with authority over the matrilineage's health and fertility. Like the creator *virigefolo*, they entail prescriptions and taboos, via divination, for the individual that they have chosen. Since they are very irritable, they require permanent attention, wearing of their insignia. One day ill-fortune strikes, an illness leads a patient to consult a diviner whose interpretation would point to the twins this time. They were offended and sent the "black figure" / *yewuo*, an abnormal state characterized by premature deaths, strange events, omens, that precisely require consultation of a diviner. We can see the importance of individual or group perception that will decide and name the threshold and the state which once reached make an interpretation inevitable, even if, as everywhere else, there is a certain code of what is to be considered as an omen, what is acceptable ("normal") and what is not. The place of *agent* of ill-fortune, occupied by the creator and the twins, can also be taken up by the fifth causal category: the ancestors of the matrilineage, *kubele*, of whom the twins are sometimes regarded as a particular avatar.

As in a number of African societies, the lineal ancestors watch over their descendants. Like the entities that were mentioned earlier on, they can have affects and intentions and they can be the source of several ills for those who neglect their sacrifices. The "spirits" of the land and of the bush / *madebele*, the original "mystic" owners of the territory where the village community settled, are also possible agents of illness and ill-fortune. Often they appear in the form of events and enigmatic encounters in the fields, of fainting fits or sudden pains, when they are annoyed because not enough respect is shown towards them, or quite simply when they "love" and pick someone out. Like the previous agents, the *madebele* manifest themselves only in this way and like the *virigefolo*, their advent is not even the outcome of a human act. The creator necessarily reveals himself one day, the *madebele* address themselves to someone without his behaviour necessarily providing a motive. In such connections human action, good or bad, legitimate or transgressive, is not indispensable for the process of causality to work. Unfortunately, it is not enough to respect the many prescriptions of each entity scrupulously to avoid ill-fortune. There is always some cause that can be invoked. However, a negative social attitude increases *a fortiori* the probability of ill-fortune and triggers off the process.

Owing to this relative maladjustment of representations and social conduct, these explanatory models cater for all possible events. Since they do not necessarily rely on real action, their validity cannot be questioned. And when they are linked to a behaviour that has indeed been adopted, they create an appropriate framework for standard social conduct, a fact largely developed by functionalist analyses. Illness is not simply the result of unpredictable whims of non-human agents or of determinist processes (mechanical factor, transgression of a taboo). What is more, illness can be a punishment for social misbehaviour. Therefore, these causal connections form a powerful and emotionally charged means of explanation. You cannot simply neglect the prescription of an ancestor, or of twins, or of the lineal power *sandoho*, if you run the risk of catching "hot body" or of your children dying.

Other causal categories, witchcraft and sorcery, can rightly be considered as a means of exercising social control. The invisible sorcerer *deo*, who deploys his evil power mainly within his matrilineage and his residence group according to the web of authority and heritage following a schema that is frequent in African societies, is often said to take advantage of an individual's misconduct to attack him, as if his behaviour made him more susceptible to ill-fortune and to illness.

The same applies to "magic" objects, cult or protecting "fetishes", *yasungyi* and *katyengele*, which are supposed to attack and defend themselves against what is conceived as a potential enemy. The malevolence of others in the form of lineal witchcraft or of aggression by magical forces is here a very meaningful aetiological framework. One could almost say that all ills can "in the end" be attributed to it, the agent-sorcerer or fetish being a sort of accelerator for the process which will end in illness or in death.

This last scheme clearly shows that these causal categories are first of all a vision of the social universe, based on the mode of circularity and of retrospective reasoning. On the one hand, by indicating an agonistic conception of social relations, a "war by all against all", where everyone defends himself to avoid being attacked and vice versa, the world of the witch and the sorcerer, correlative of the world of counter-sorcerers, "owners of fetishes" or institutionalized healers, can afterwards explain all the events according to the "force" and hence the victory of the one or the other. For instance, the illness *meheni*/hook, which is a disease "thrown" by the enemy in the form of an invisible hook in the food of the victim, will be cured if the therapist, who structurally participates in the world of witchcraft to combat the disease, is more powerful than the aggressor and if he did not strike a deal with him at the expense of the victim. Otherwise, the outcome will be disastrous.

On the other hand, imputing sorcery, attributing any ailment to a causality of this type, also follows a circular reasoning pattern, ultimately always depending on a social consensus, as we can see from the above-mentioned notions of *tete* and *toro*, indicating a destiny of ill-fortune and a life of misfortune. For instance, a sterile woman is said to be *tetefolo*, bearer of such a destiny. A common explanation is that sterility is due to an evil instrumental action of a sorcerer. However, the woman herself can also be considered as the sorceress who may have sacrificed her entire future offspring to the invisible association of sorcerers. She is then the object and agent of the aggression at the same time. Although sterility is held to be a great ill-fortune, sterile women are feared and laughed at. The social meaning of ill-fate can therefore always be reversed, reassessed, and consequently also the causality connected to it, according to extrinsic criteria. What is the social position of the "old woman" in her kin group? Who are all the dependents of that "old man"? Who is afraid of him? Since normally no one is so foolish as to declare himself a sorcerer, an invisible and necessary explanatory principle, the signs that prove his existence also have to do with an ever irrefutable or "infalsifiable", as Popper would say, retrospective judgment. The sorcerer is the one who is too handsome, too ugly, too poor, too lucky or too unlucky....

Before describing the ninth causal category, that of *yawige*, a feature common to the a priori explicative configurations has to be pointed out; they trace, at the same time, one-to-one, preferential and multireferential connections. Some symptoms or ill-fortunes, some abnormal events or omens, refer a priori to precise instances. For example, coughs or scabies are supposed to "indicate" the intervention of the creator. The same applies to diseases of the mouth and the stomach, where the transgression of a taboo is the intermediate operator. Illnesses with an uncertain or fatal outcome, such as the "interior abscess"/*fungo funingi* where the sick person dies suddenly without having previously suffered from any apparent symptoms, are preferably connected to the action of a sorcerer, *debele*. Leprosy, *yanyemi*/"red disease", is thus connected to sorcery. Depending on the symptoms, and therefore on their social recognition, it can be regarded either as the effect of the "spell"/*wa* of an evil enemy, or as a sign of the patient's duplicity and his membership of the world of sorcerers.

However, these apparently one-to-one connections, where such and such a cause is a priori supposed to bring about such and such an effect, can be misleading, because all the illnesses can in fact be linked to more than one instance, as these few examples suggest. The peculiarities of a symptom are not enough to indicate that it has one single cause. Sudden fainting, for example, may just as well indicate the action of spirits of the land/*madebele* as the action of a sorcerer, who can also manifest himself a priori through such signs. It is precisely the variable and loose nature of the nosological categories that make it possible to move from one cause to another when practical reasons so demand. The importance of the metaphorizations typical of the Fodonon representations should not be neglected, however, since they give a meaning to these preferential links: conceptions of the body, the inside and the outside for sorcery, metaphors of the fall, of the bringing down for the action of spirits that "fall" on their victim or "catch" him, etc., flowing from the symbolic qualities of these entities.

Nevertheless, from the point of view of a priori causality, most symptoms can be connected to many interchangeable aetiologies, following the actual development of the pathological process. Common syndromes, such as diarrhoea, oedemas, rheumatism, "stomach-aches" and, above all, the already-mentioned "hot body"/ *tyefuru*, can in fact refer to all the possible causal categories.

Here we recognize the bundle of interchangeable causes which for R. Horton[14] characterized traditional causal thought, which ascribes a contemporary plurality of possible antecedents to an effect, in the inclusive disjunction mode "either... or..." Stomach-aches can be due to either the transgression of a sexual taboo, or to an object "cast" in sorcery, etc. This flexibility permits precisely for what Horton calls "secondary elaboration". If a causal connection is inadequate, obsolete or contradicted by experience, it is "re-worked" to acquire a higher explicative value. The theoretical framework, the causal categories, remains. The blame for any failure to explain and foresee the event is laid on defective human actions, mainly misinterpretation or bad performance of the therapeutic ritual, incompetence or weakness of the diviner or therapist, or the transgression of relevant taboos.

So it is that the causal category *yawige* occupies a peculiar position in the causality charts. It provides a comparatively constant link, both for a priori interpretations and for actual illness situations which, contrary to Horton's belief, are not freely interchangeable with all the other causes. Closely linked to the theory of taboos/ *yafungo*, the illnesses of *yawige*, "thing that pursues", are children's diseases that present specific signs. They are imputed to eating, seeing or touching, through the mother or an ancestor of the sick child, an animal either living or dead, or to the killing of this animal during the hunt by the father while his wife was pregnant. These acts are taboo for the mother. The the operator is the animal's *nyuma*. It is common to all living beings and is "emitted" by all dead bodies in the bush, which are capable of "catching"/ *tyo* the individuals with whom they are in contact.

When a child displays these symptoms, it is immediately deduced, and divination is unnecessary here, that the conduct of the ascendants is involved and that such or such an animal has "caught" the child. For example, *pyenge we tyo*/"the hare caught him", is the name of an illness where a child sleeps with his eyes open, he cannot fall asleep "like the hare at night sleeping with his eyes open"; and *fo*/python, is the name of an illness where the child drools, opens its mouth "like a python" and sleeps constantly. Examples abound, almost every animal, whether domestic or wild, can be an agent of these illnesses. This schema of causality, which we have dealt with very briefly, is interesting for two reasons apart from the metaphoric and metonymic operations that it offers.

On the one hand, it is a particular form of causality, based on the idea of contagion, that differs from the reasoning involved in the preceding categories: ancestors, spirits, ... It shows the heterogeneity of the traditional structures of causality. Like the preceding categories, it refers to a general theory, of the matrilineage in this case, concerning procreative relations, the role of the father, time and space.

On the other hand, the notion of *yawige*/thing that pursues, indicates not only a content, illnesses sent by animals, but also a way of action that can be joined to other agents that are causal categories. The creator, ancestors, spirits, twins and the *sandoho* power of the matrilineage can all "pursue" individuals and be said to be agents of *yawige*, which in this case means "contamination". Such a polysemy allowing a causal category to stand as content on its own, but to specify, as a form, the other possible categories, illustrates the structural impossibility of working out taxonomies, and the logical paradoxes of the theories of causation. However, this is not necessarily illogical or inconsistent; the paradox emerges only in an overall systematic view of traditional theories. If they are taken for what they are, i.e., "local" explanations (in theory) valid in practical situations, the paradox disappears.

The notion of taboo/*yafungo*, ever present in Fodonon representations, is in this aspect similar to the notion of *yawige*. A transgression is very frequently mentioned a priori in the explanation of ill-fortune, on a one-to-one basis. Every transgression is assumed to bring about ill-fortune and illness for the transgressor or for one of the members of his kinship. Inversely, many ills are readily deciphered, by divination, as the transgression, known or unknown, of a taboo. *Yafungo*/the taboo, is a quality that can be applied to any object, status, function, circumstance, moment, living being, etc. It is a "positive" quality of the substance or the action. Thus people say that it is the *yafungo* of a certain matriclan to eat guib, on pain of illness. The important thing is that this notion is at the same time an autonomous factor of ill-fortune and can be attributed to all the forces mentioned above, ancestors, creator, etc. These are then the agents and the taboo is the "reason" for the illness-penalty and its being triggered off. For example, the creator *yirigefolo* can forbid his protege to eat gombo sauce. If he eats it, he does so at his own risk, especially if he had been warned of the danger by divination. He could then get *nyofo-rigi*/"flayed mouth".

Leaving aside for the time being the last possible a priori causal category, the *sandoho* force of the matrilineage, we can close this short description of the first register of coherence, the framework of the explanation, with a summary of its principal aspects. It forms a "finite" structure to which an infinite number of fortunate or unfortunate events can be related. It cannot be constituted as a taxonomy, since the actual choices depend on a practical logic. It refers to a theory of the physical world which, unlike a scientific theory, cannot be refuted, because it emphasizes causal reasoning of a circular nature. It is an extension of the theory of the physical universe *and* of the social relationships (lineage, land) between man and that universe and among men themselves.

2. The Two Other Registers of Coherence: Effective Interpretation of Divination and Therapy

For the Fodonon, the particular interpretation of a disorder belongs to a different register than the representations which each one makes a priori of the event. It is an a posteriori exercise of causality. It is possible that a disorder may not be interpreted; one can wait for it to end or immediately resort to therapy. Most often an explanation is called for. The victim and those around him may spontaneously provide one, but more often than not divinatory institutions take charge of interpretations. Depending on their structures, they refer to certain preferred causal categories, and the causality depends largely on the *initial choice*, by the patient or his relatives, spouse or members of his lineage, of such an institution. Indeed, if recourse is had to an "owner of fetishes"/*yasungofolo* or a *nikmo*/"root hitter", who generally exercise the functions both of diviner and "professional" therapist, or to a healer/*nookarga*/"he who changes into a buffalo", who specializes in accidents and different traumas, the causality will very probably lie in sorcery and evil aggression of a magic nature, because of the typical conceptions of ill-fortune of these institutions. They are agonistic conceptions of the world of sorcerers and counter-sorcerers, where victory belongs to the "strongest"/*gba*. The therapy, applied by those who interpret, is governed by the causality chosen.

However, if the *sandoho*, the favourite form of Senufo divination, is called in, as happens most frequently, people consult for the slightest abnormal event, then the appropriate connection will be selected from all the causal categories previously listed. *Sandoho* divination is an institution that is normally concerned only with interpretation. It does not provide any instructions for therapy (remedies, for example).

Conversely, the therapeutic register forms a third register of coherence. The "common" therapists, *katyao* or *sityilio*, owners of "leaves"/*were*, of remedy ingredients, who have a certain knowledge about pharmacopoeia, do not let their therapies depend on the cause of their clients' afflictions. One and the same remedy can be used to treat all the patients indiscriminately, or it can be special for one particular syndrome such as coughs, headaches, etc. The administration of *were* remedies, objects endowed with the powers and support of specific taboos that guarantee their efficacity, follow criteria completely different from divination. A sick person can directly consult either a therapist who "owns" *were* and who has a reputation or a divineress, or both, in which order does not matter. The interpretation need not necessarily precede the therapy. The register of effective interpretation and of therapy, therefore, appears to be relatively *closed* in this society.[15]

The *sandoho* institution, which is too complex to be described in great detail,[16] provides a structure for the causal categories listed above and, at the same time, it singles out from among the possibilities a unique causal and prescriptive course at a given moment. The following are its main features:

On the one hand, it is a *divinatory institution*. The divineress disposes of precisely the finite series of categories, God, twins..., represented by objects-emblems, and of no others. The interpretation of the configurations formed by these objects, when they have been thrown on the ground, is followed by the progressive determination of a causality for the client, by means of the interplay of questions with binary answers that the divineress asks and repeats to her *madebele* spirits. After the divineress has indicated a single cause in view of what has happened before, the client, who remains quiet at first, can discuss and, if necessary, adjust this interpretation, if it does not fit in with the reasons for his visit. For example, a child of the client has fallen ill, because a member of his matrilineage has forgotten to keep the promise to make a sacrifice which he had made to the lineal "fetishes" before the child was born. Some diagnoses refer to past events and categories that are invisible, for instance, to the fact that a child is ill because he has been taken by an illness of *yawige* contracted by his mother during pregnancy. Others, referring to empirical facts, can be challenged by the client. For instance, the promise of a sacrifice mentioned above may well never have been made. Again, a conflict between the real events and the framework of causality, which does not call the latter into question, is explained retrospectively as human fallibility. The diviner may be considered incompetent, or he may have transgressed the taboos of his profession.

On the other hand, the *sandoho* institution is the "power" of every matrilineage, the guarantor of its fertility and continuity. From that point of view it is the paradigm of all causal categories. They are all described in the lineal theory as entities which have previously entered into an alliance with an ancestor and are conserved as the "mystical" inheritance of the lineage: such are twins, lineage fetishes, water spirits.... All these entities, then, describe the physical universe and they are also inscriptions which are present in every lineage. The general structure of ill-fortune is thus conceived as the effect, the reactivation of instances which are pre-inscribed, "already present", in the symbolic history of the lineage.

This power is in fact also a possible cause independent ill-fortune. A series of children's diseases, "hot body" in particular, women's diseases, the ill-fortune and conflicts which have built up within the lineage, are readily decoded by divination as an effect of the *sandoho* for two reasons: either because this power requires continuity in the lineage of the filial "chain" of women "attached" to its altar, or because it is the agent of punishment for its principal taboo, namely the illicit sexual relations of the women of the lineage. The solution to the perceived afflictions depend on this "attachment", which takes the form of female initiation at every generation. These women, who guarantee the continuity of the lineage, have to bear many, very restrictive taboos.

This force is, therefore, at the same time a *cause* and a *means* of resolution of the symptom, as considered within the framework of the lineage. This feature can also be found in other African societies, for example, in cult or therapy associations set up by former victims of the ill-fortune. Like other categories, this power forms the link between the social order and the explanation of ill-fortune, because it assumes at the same time an explanatory function and one of support for the lineal order. It may be the intermediary for the transgression of social rules to be connected to the illness, since its role is to represent the values and the ethic of the lineage and it has the power to send the illness. This is true of the other causal categories, ancestors, spirits, ..., which are both representations in the Durkheimian sense of the word, and agents endowed with intentions and power with a social function and a cognitive (explanatory) role.

We can, therefore, apply the term *circularity* to one of the rules that organize the schema of causality of the Fodonon society; it is like an enclosure around possible models, which are always true, always confirmed by experience, as illustrated by the theory of sorcery. Divination works only with the categories listed, even if it proposes connections with infinite content. The conception of circularity is not a proof of intellectual incapacity, it is an aspect of the theory and of the actual functioning of lineage organization, the lineage as a combination of forces and a continuous kinship that is trying to keep its numbers as high as possible. Causality founds its own coherence, just as interpretation has its own, which is governed by the demands of practical adjustments to real life, which, though informed by a priori causality, are not intended to call it into question.

Therapeutics, however, relies on a great capacity of assimilation, of openness towards foreign elements, from Islam or biomedicine, for example, because it is not an application of causality which is not assessed according to criteria of therapeutic efficacity. The relative impermeability among the registers of interpretation and of the resolution of ill-fortune ensures that the multiplication of therapeutic alternatives ("medical pluralism") does not lead to changes in the traditional explanatory model. The (recognized) efficacity of Western biomedicine does not affect causal thought, because its primary function is precisely to explain, not to heal.

Ill-fortune, therefore, is the point where at least three universes of connected, but distinct, coherent representations, converge. This is why changes in this society today result, from time to time, in a rejection of all the traditional schema of causality, especially that of the lineage *sandoho*, or, in earlier days, in the adoption of prophetic cults and, today, the conversion to Christianity, which is asked to: "Deliver us from taboos".... Abandoning these schema is done by breaking away, substituting one conception of the world for another unlike in other, perhaps more "open", African societies that have more easily juxtaposed the old and the new gods.

NOTES

1. E.E. Evans-Pritchard, *Witchcraft, Oracles, and Magic Among the Azande*, Oxford, 1937. C. Levi-Strauss, *La pensée sauvage*, Plon, Paris, 1962. V. Turner, *The Drums of Affliction*, Clarendon Press, Oxford, 1968; and *The Ritual Process*, Aldine, Chicago, 1969; and "A Ndembu Doctor in Practice", re-

printed in *Magic, Faith and Healing*, A. Kiev ed., Glencoe: Free press, New York, 1964.

2. M. Gluckman, *The Allocation of Responsibility*, Manchester, Manchester University Press, 1972.

3. *Prophétisme et Thérapeutique*, edited by C. Piault, Paris, Hermann, 1975.

4. G. Lewis, *Knowledge of Illness in a Sepik Society: the Study of the Gnau, New Guinea*, London, The Athlone Press, 1975. J.B. Loudon ed. *Social Anthropology and Medicine*, London, Academic Press, 1976. A. Young, "Some Implications of Medical Beliefs and Practices for Social Anthropology", *American Anthropologist*, 78, 1976, pp. 5-24.

5. A. Kleinman, *Patients and Healers in the Context of Culture*, Berkeley, University of California Press, 1980.

6. G.M. Foster, "Disease Etiologies in Non-Western Medical Systems", *American Anthropologist*, 78, 4, December 1976, pp. 773-782.

7. T. Kuhn, *The Structure of Scientific Revolutions*, 2nd edition, Chicago, University of Chicago Press, 1962.

8. A. Young, art. cit., p. 6.

9. J.Goody, *The Domestication of the Savage Mind*, Cambridge, 1977.

10. J. Skorupski, *Symbol and Theory, a Philosophic Study of Theories or Religion in Social Anthropology*, Cambridge, Cambridge University Press, 1976.

11. R. Horton, "African Traditional Thought and Western Science", *Africa*, XXXVII, 1-2, pp.50-71 and 155-187; and "Tradition and Modernity Revisited", in *Rationality and Relativism*, M. Hollis and S. Lukes eds, Oford, B. Blackwell, 1982.

12. This table is based on the material of an article by N. Sindzingre and A. Zempleni, "Réflexions sur la causalité de la maladie chez les Senufo de Côte d'Ivoire", *Social Science and Medicine*, vol 15 B, 1981, pp. 279-293.

13. E.E. Evans-Pritchard, *Essays in Social Anthropology*.

14. R. Horton, art. cit., p. 169 sq.

15. These features are explained in: N. Sindzingre, "Healing is what healing does: pragmatic resolution of misfortune among the Senufo (Ivory Coast)", in Healing Paths, M. Augé ed., *History and Anthropology*, Harwood Academic Publishers, forthcoming.

16. This notion was developed in a doctorate thesis on related subjects: N. Sindzingre, *Organisation lignagère et représentations de la maladie chez les Fodonon, Senufo de Côte d'Ivoire*, Paris, EHESS, 1981.

Chapter 3

STERILITY, ARIDITY, DROUGHT: SOME INVARIANTS OF SYMBOLIC THOUGHT

F. Héritier

Arid, adj. (Lat. *aridus*). Dry, sterile: arid land. Fig. arid mind: that cannot produce anything. Arid subject: that does not lend itself to developments. Ant. humid, fertile.

Sterility... Apart from a man or a woman's personal sterility, there are cases where sterility cannot be attributed to either partner, but to their union, and where both prove to be fertile with another partner.

LAROUSSE UNIVERSEL

If an author is fertile, then his writings flow. His texts are full of ideas. He may even be extremely knowledgeable about his subject, or suffer from logorrhea. But when he has nothing more to say or to write about, he dries up, his mind is arid, his imagination runs dry. Immediately the phraseology of social judgment tends to use images opposing mainly humidity or fertile humours to sterile aridness. Nevertheless, it is not so much a mere metaphorical transposition of one domain (nature) to another (verbal creations of the mind), as an emphasis on the *same sensitive properties* of things and facts of a different nature, by using shared terms. In short, they are the odd expressions drawn from a set of collective representations that derive their truth from the perception of a visible, obvious particularity that, in broad terms, could be stated as follows: flows of all kinds are necessary for the production of all life. In our culture, it would be comparatively easy to show from this standpoint that the interpretations of fertility and sterility spring, at least as far as language is concerned, both from a symbolic system of representations that establish a relationship between the course of the natural world and its reproduction, the human person in his flesh and in his mind, as well as the interplay of social rules, as if it were the most natural thing to do. Jean Starobinski's recently published study on chlorosis contains an excellent example of these connections.[1]

We are interested here in sterility of the body, and not in sterility of the mind, and in how it is perceived in "primitive", "exotic" and unlettered societies. The apparently diverse beliefs about sterility depend, of course, for each group of people, on its own ideological construction of representations, a perfectly autonomous coherent structure. Examining a certain number of data, nevertheless, suggests that it is possible to relate certain specific ethnic conceptions encountered to one or more universal sets of invariants that bring out their common logic. In so doing, we remain faithful to Durkheim's approach. He believed that "thinking in conceptions is not simply isolating and grouping the features common to a certain number of objects, it is subsuming variable elements under a classification of permanent characteristics."[2] From the outset, three sets of characteristics appear. A statement of the first two should not a priori give rise to many objections:

The discourse on sterility, though it is always based on concrete observations, is founded neither on a scientific knowledge of physiology, nor on morality. It is a discourse on social practice and the rules of conduct related to it.

Sterility is always and everywhere automatically understood to be feminine. It clearly stresses something about the social relation between the sexes.

The discourse on the causes of sterility, as well as one the (generally implicit) reasons for fertility, expresses a homology between the nature of the world, the human body, and society, and the possibility of transferring elements from one register to another. This homology expresses itself in variable symbolic contents, but according to identical formal laws. We shall try here to unravel the threads of one of the contents which seems to re-occur very frequently.

The representations of sterility are always based on precise, concrete observations, and not on a corpus of scientifically recognized abstract knowledge, and the interpretation grids of this phenomenon refer to social practice. The recently learned explanation of the fundamental mechanisms of gametogenesis and impregnation has very little to do with it, either in our modern popular beliefs or in our former beliefs or with the current beliefs of other peoples. For want of a scientifically proved explanation, and it is important to remember, to paraphrase Durkheim (op. cit. p. 625), that if it is to be believed, it is not enough for it to be true it has to be in line with other beliefs, the learned discourse naturally refers to social practice as the only interpretive system possible. Nothing is more instructive on this subject than the chapter Verrier Elwin[3] devotes to the problem of adolescent sterility, and especially sterility in the *gothul*, the house for young people of the Muria Indian tribe. This is a school for pre-matrimonial social and sexual education with many partners. Many other populations have similar institutions. We now know that over a variable period of time, which may last some few years, after menarche, not all menstrual cycles are accompanied by ovulation.[4] The number of anovulatory cycles depends, of course, on the individual and it diminishes with time. During this period, young women enjoy a certain natural protection against the danger of impregnation. Indeed, from the beginning of this century, several authors had noticed how few young girls became pregnant in the many societies that tolerated or advocated pre-conjugal sexual freedom, often within different types of special institutions encouraging it: houses for youngsters, bachelors' houses, common dormitories (*bukumatula* of the Trobrianders, *ghotul* of the Muria, *manyatta* of the Masai, *agamang* of the Ifugao, etc.) However, there was no evidence of particularly effective contraception or abortion techniques, nor of a surprisingly high number of abortions or infanticides. Malinowski has raised the following question: "Can there be a physiological law that reduces the chances of conception, when a woman engages in sexual activity at an early age, has an uninterrupted sexual life and often changes lovers?"[5] The answers to this question (which in itself provides the elements for a socially founded answer) that Elwin proposes are striking, because they correspond to nothing else but a literary, rational and clever structure for widespread beliefs. According to Barton, it is the intensity of sexual activity during adolescence that causes sterility, by maintaining a state of hyperaemia of the female organs.[6] For Rentoul, the Trobrianders had "a special capacity or privilege to expel the male semen to which they could resort after every coitus."[7] In his *Medical History of Contraception*, N.E. Himes repeats this idea.[8] According to G.H.L. Pitt-Rivers, "sterility as a result of promiscuity is due to the mixture of sperm of different men."[9] For Seligman, who also believed that "young Papuan women conceived less easily than white women", this point of view is reaffirmed by the Sinangolo belief that a single coitus cannot cause impregnation and that very regular sexual intercourse during at least one month is required for impregnation to take place.[10] And then there is also the belief, which is, nevertheless, expressed with doubt, nuance and reservation, that the woman's passiveness and lack of enjoyment can be accompanied by a certain control of uterine reflexes that reduce the possibility of impregnation.

Women's different racial aptitude, too regular or, on the contrary, too irregular intercourse, sex at an early age, too many male partners, an idea which in itself implies a surprising double hypothesis: prolonged impregnation without fertilization and the encounter of antagonistic sperm that annihilate one another, are all rationalizations of a certain idea about sexual practice. All in all, the Muria, who claim that, under the influence of a deity, young women are protected in the *ghotul* from conception during three years after their menarche, are closest to the truth. As Verrier Elwin said: "There must be centuries of observation behind this faith in a sterile interval." (p. 292.)

These judgments, which we believe offer many normative standpoints, translate, indeed, a certain idea of the cause-effect relationship that would exist between a biological evolution and social rules. In this case, the practice of "de-regulated" sex, from the point of view of the observer of course, that is to say, from the point of view of the social norm which he holds, copulating too often, too early, with too many different partners, has sterilizing effects. However, in the societies in question these same reasons will, in the same cause-effect relationship, be used in a positive sense this time, namely to found a socially "regulated" sexual practice for adolescents. It is also because they believe that one single act of intercourse cannot bring about conception, but that regular and prolonged intercourse with the same partner is required, that, in the *ghotul*, couples who are together for a long time cannot have complete sexual intercourse too often, or that evening partners can have intercourse freely as long as they change partner every night. From the Muria standpoint "pregnancy demands at the same time psychological and physical concentration on being faithful to one partner", says V. Elwin (p. 161), that is why it is typical of matrimony.

The same faith in a sterile interval during adolescence and subject to regulated sexual practice exists, in word and in deed, in populations other than the Muria. It is perfectly possible to allow or encourage adolescents to have sexual relations and at the same time rebuke them if the young woman becomes pregnant when she should not and when their status does not permit it, because the pregnancy implies *ipso facto* that they did not respect the correlative rules of sexual practice. But it is sometimes surprising to hear informants give reasons why it is not only the mystical entities comforted by codified sexual practice that bring about this protection. They exist alongside or are based on adequate physiological back-up, identified as responsible by precise and concrete observations. The Azande think that a child is the result of a fusion, of undetermined nature, between male sperm and female mucus that both contain *mbisimo, "children souls", granted by God, who also allows the meeting during the sexual act.*[11] The child will be a boy or a girl depending on whether the male or the female principle is stronger during this encounter. If one of the two partners has no *mbisimo*, the union will be fruitless. However, Evans-Pritchard adds (pp. 402, 403) that it is only upon maturity that God grants these "children souls" and that the individual becomes fertile. Before maturity, the sperm of young men is as clear as water. It is "simply urine", they say. It becomes loaded with "children souls" only when it thickens and looks like egg-white, that is to say, rarely before the age of 17, according to the Azande. It is also only after their full physical development that the mucus produced by young women thickens and also contains "children souls" given by God. Actually, many men do not worry at the beginning if their young spouses do not become pregnant, and sometimes they do not even start worrying until the women's breasts are sagging and it is no longer possible to claim that they are not yet fully developed.

In these discourses on adolescent sterility and, therefore, ironically, also on the normal conditions for fertility within marriage, there are no major disagreements between the observers and the observed. The same causal interpretation, which in neither case is founded on sound knowledge of the physiological mechanisms in question, shows in fact the close relation of parallels that exist between a social norm or practice and an individual corporal reality. The only exception is that the points of view of the observers mentioned above include, in the very terms they used, a kind of ethical judgment (of which one may legitimately think that it expresses the moral norms of their own societies in terms of what is good and bad), whereas the others did not do this. Not all primitive societies advocate sexual freedom before marriage. On the contrary. But whether they recommend it or not, it is striking to observe how few strictly moral appreciations of the presumed causes of sterility there are, even if within marriage it is believed to be the effect of adultery or evil, female practices to prevent conception. A sterile woman is often looked down on, because she is a totally deficient, incomplete, unfinished being. Sometimes she is replaced by another spouse given by her own family, if her husband has paid considerable matrimonial compensation for her, as is the case among the Lovedu,[12] the Thonga,[13] and the Azande. A woman who is really sterile, not simply a woman whose children are stillborn, may sometimes be considered as responsible for her destiny because of acts of transgression which she is thought to have committed either voluntarily or involuntarily and of which sterility is the signifying stigma. As we shall see later on, she can even be made to suffer the consequences in society, in particular when sterility is synonymous with sorcery. The Ojibwa, for instance, who hold that a fruitless marriage is always due to the wife's deficiency,[14] justify this imputation by explaining that the woman has (perhaps against her wishes or even simply without being aware of it) been united in a dream with the people around her (p. 37). She can even be made to suffer the consequences in society after her death. Rattray tells how Ashanti men or women who die childless have the soles of their feet pierced with long thorns before being buried. The body is told why it is treated so badly: "You did not engender, or bear, a child; do not come back to behave like that again."[15] In a few regions of Samoa, the sterile woman who had never menstruated and who was presumed to have no womb was buried after having the small of her back thrust through with a sharp stick to let the blood flow that she had never lost.[16] The image of the sterile woman is that of a humiliated, vexed victim, who is judged responsible and who is even accused of sorcery, but who is never morally guilty.

Sterility is regarded, however, as only a feminine problem. Most ethnological literature on the subject ignores the existence of specific male sterility, not so much because the authors have always applied their own cultural presuppositions to the information that they collected, but because the information was formulated in such a way by the informants themselves. However, it seems that the result would probably have been roughly the same either way. There are good, obvious, common sense reasons to explain this, since the biological facts which are used as a basis are immediately perceptible and are part of a universal corpus of observations on human nature that every society makes. It is the woman who bears children, gives birth to them, nurtures them, during a fertile period which has a visible beginning, menarche, and an end, menopause. If a woman did not become pregnant during that period of her life, then that can only be due to her own nature, if the schema of comprehension and interpretation of the facts are applied which do not take into account the bio-chemical nature of conception, when they do take into account the necessary, if not sufficient, link between copulation and procreation.

This ignorance was also ours until the end of the 17th century, since it was only between 1672 and 1677 that de Graaf and Leeuwenhoek respectively discovered the female ovum and the existence of sperm in semen. However, these discoveries on their own were not enough to settle the question of the conception process scientifically. A fierce debate continued for almost a century between thinkers and scholars to determine which of the two was solely responsible for the genesis of the embryo, the ovum, where the germs of all future offspring were already formed, or the sperm, moved by animalcules that would find the sustenance necessary for their development on a neutral terrain.

It is, moreover, very likely that an analysis of the notion of fertility / sterility, in our culture in different eras, based on scholarly, demographic and medical studies, would show the same ideological prevalence of the woman's responsibility for sterility, and not only as a simple popular belief. Only recently, for instance, has medical research been systematically carried out into the man's responsibility, which would actually be at the source of 30% to 40% of sterility in couples. In the remarkable work that Frank Lorimer together with other authors has devoted to the influence of culture on human fertility, it can easily be observed that the figures regarding couples always refer to the woman.[17] However, a worrisome issue remains. F. Lorimer remarks (p. 49) with regard to the difference in fecundity in the life cycle: "Questions relating to the maturation and decline of fertility have been discussed here solely with reference to women. Comparable processes take place in the lives of men, but over a much longer span. In any case, advance in the age of one spouse is linked with that of the other. If we recognize that apparent decline in fecundity in women with advancing age may be in part a function of declining fecundity in men, or in the conjugal relations of spouses, we can ignore these aspects in order to simplify the analysis." So, for the decline of fecundity as well as for complete sterility, the idea is the same in demography as it is in anthropology: the male factor can be ignored.

Naturally, male impotence is recognized everywhere, but in general it is the only case in which the man is blamed for the couple's infertility. Hence, among the Fanti, the wife's relatives will encourage her to leave her husband if after six months there is still no sign of any children being on the way, for every woman must have children to enlarge the lineage, since the Fanti are a matrilineal society. It is the husband who is blamed for this failure in the first place, "unless he has already demonstrated his potency", says Christiansen.[18] What is questioned is his potency, not his fecundity. Similarly, among their Ashanti neighbours, who are also a matrilineal community, where a childless couple is mocked, (both the husband and wife), the husband is coarsely nicknamed "wax penis"

(Rattray, op. cit., p. 67) and because of his flaccidity he is thus blamed
for the absence of progeny. However, in patrilineal societies there are
often compensatory mechanisms thanks to which male impotence and
a fortiori sterility (if the two concepts can be clearly distinguished) are of
no importance as such, because of the social distinction that is established between social (pater) paternity and physical (reproductive) paternity. Among the Samo, as in many other West African societies, a
young woman who had been promised in legitimate marriage in her
early childhood by the men of her lineage, was given to her husband
after giving birth to her first child. But this first child, of whom the
husband was the socially recognized father, was in fact the natural child
of another man, a pre-marital partner, chosen by the young woman
herself or by her mother, who was closer to her age and more to her liking
than her legitimate husband. The young people had lived together
completely legitimately and openly at night only, after the girl's father
had made the puberty sacrifice for her, otherwise she would not have
been able to have sexual relations without risking imminent punishment
(she would waste away). These pre-nuptial amorous relations end at the
birth of the first child, when the wife joins her husband, the social father
of the child, or after three years if this union remains fruitless. So, save
in this specific case where after three years the wife joins her husband
even without having given birth to a child, a man can have at least as
many children as he has legitimate spouses, if the children survive.
Moreover, the other children that these legitimate wives might have
from extra-marital affairs, or during the husband's prolonged absence,
rightfully belong to him, if with the intimidation tactics at his disposal
he can lure his wife and the children born in the meantime back to him.
It also happens that if a marriage is fruitless, a wife who is very attached
to her husband, agrees with him, admittedly not without a certain
duplicity, to pretend to leave him and then come back to him when she
is pregnant, thus granting him, with the help of a deceived second
husband, the social paternity he needs. Everything revolves around
social paternity. However, for the patrilineage to survive and the cult of
the ancestors to be continued from generation to generation without
interruption, it is not even necessary for a man to have children in his
name. If his brothers have offspring and he calls them "my children",
then after his death they will worship him and pay him the respect due
to the ancestors of the lineage. And the component of his person, the
spirit (*yiri*), which returns after his death to leave his mark in a newly
born boy of the lineage, can return in the son or grandson of a brother as
well as his own grandson. For women this is not the case. A woman's

double who is in distress and demands specific sacrifices after death, can only be heard by her own female descendants and her spirit can return only in her own grandchildren. If she bears no children, she might just as well never have existed.[19]

Audrey Richard describes a very similar situation among the Haya, a Bantu population of the Interlacustrian Kingdoms. There can be no illegitimate children without a social father in their community either. The social father of a yet unborn child is the man with whom the mother had her first sexual relation after having recovered from the previous childbirth. A. Richards explains that this right to the first-born child was granted to the husband by rituals when the marriage was consummated and that they must later be repeated after each childbirth.[20] In a way, the situation is completely opposite to that among the Samo, since marriage does not give the husband all the rights over the children to come, but the result is the same. A man who is sterile and even impotent can thus obtain the heir that he so desperately wants. Indeed, as the author explicitly indicates, a man can work out a plan to acquire the paternity he lacks. He has to come to an agreement, in one way or another, with a fertile woman, so that she grants, or pretends to have granted, her first *post-partum* relation to him ("it is her sole right to state which man has had access to her after delivery", p. 376). Thus, the next child she gives birth to shall be his. Consequently, it is perfectly possible, as with the Samo, that a man who himself has never procreated is the legal father of several children. Very often, however, these children, who are called *bisisi*, are the first-born children of subsequent marriages who are given to the previous husband who had the initial ritual right or who acquired it by means of a *post-partum* first relation.

Nevertheless, the question of the spouses' respective responsibility for the sterility of the couple may take on slightly different forms, depending on the views on conception and the development of the child in the mother's womb. As can be expected, there is indeed an obvious contiguity between the ideas on fecundation and gestation and those on sterility. To appreciate them at their true value, an inventory of paradigmatic archetypes should be drawn up based on the documentation available. Such an inventory remains to be made. In general, if conception is not attributed to spiritual causes alone, it is supposed to result from a relation between two "waters" or between two bloods. The paternal blood is carried by the sperm, a classic conception that was also at the core of popular Western beliefs before, but also after, the advent of scientific knowledge of embryogenesis, since we see in marriage and in the act of procreation the union of two bloods. This encounter takes place at a favourable moment, either because of luck (the orifice of the small clot of blood that whirls round in the uterus is turned towards the vagina exactly at the moment of ejaculation, this is the Samo conception;[21] or each spouse has a snake in the abdomen carrying the reproductive function and the man's snake spits out the semen that is either accepted or rejected by the woman's, but the head has to be turned in the right direction, this is the Lovedu conception[22]), or because of a constant disposition: the Muria believe that for seven days after menstruation a little blood lingers in a low pocket of the uterus, blood that powerfully draws "the water of man" (Elwin, op. cit., p. 294). Intercourse during that period is thought to bear fruit inevitably, which explains the extra precaution taken in the *ghotul* to prohibit sexual intercourse during those days.

But, whatever the favourable time, the bloods that meet do not necessarily mix; the bloods are not on an equal footing. The matrilineal Bemba believe that only the mother's blood comes into the child's constitution, regardless of the activating nature of the sexual relations. However, the Navaho, another matrilineal society, think that children come from the man's blood. It must, however, be able to assert itself in order to mix with the woman's blood during an encounter that is regarded as an authentic struggle between opposing forces. If the man's blood is stronger, his spouse will conceive, but if it is her blood that wins, then she will not.[23] We will come back later to the basic idea behind this interesting view. In many other societies, be they matrilineal or patrilineal or even cognatic, this paternal exclusiveness exists where the mother, according to explicit metaphors, merely lends her body for the development of the foetus, like a sack that is filled or a dish in which a first-class meal is cooked.

Between these two extremes, there is a range of different compositions, where both sexes co-operate in the making of a child, either both in the same manner or each in their own way, endowing the child-to-be with some of their attributes. A Samo child has its body and bones from its mother (from its mother's blood), but its blood comes from its father (from its father's sperm). Except perhaps in those cases where a child is regarded as solely the mother's creation, it is almost always believed that regular sexual intercourse during pregnancy, or at least until the sixth or seventh month, is necessary, so that the father's semen nourishes and constitutes the foetus with essential contributions[24] or forms the foetus by gradually giving it a human shape.[25]

The very idea of questioning the respective responsibilities of the spouses for sterility might lead us to think that the chances of the balance tipping either way are equal. In fact, it is not really a matter of determining who is responsible, but rather the idea that the failure of a couple to procreate may be the result of their bloods being incapable of fusing, which we could call blood "incompatibility", an idea based again on precise, concrete observations. This idea is clearly expressed by the Samo. If a woman has no children after a few years of marriage and after having been through the appropriate propitiatory rituals, the diviners are consulted to learn the ultimate cause of this failure. Sometimes the answer is that "their bloods do not go together". In that case, and in that case only, is the separation of the couple that was united in legitimate marriage socially acceptable, without causing any offense to either family, and the young woman is authorized to try her luck with a second husband. This is by virtue of the same hypothesis, which is perhaps more bearable psychologically than other beliefs of the same society on the causes of sterility and which offers a ray of hope at least, that completely barren women are among those who have most marital experience, of up to seven or eight successive husbands. A sterile woman is a woman who "has wandered around a lot" in pursuit of a dream: finding a blood that is compatible with her own. It is also by virtue of that same hypothesis that, if she is attached to her husband and refuses to leave him, a legitimate spouse agrees with her husband to have a child from another blood for the social benefit of her husband.

This notion of blood incompatibility is found among other populations too. The matrilineal Ashanti, for example, explain procreation by the fact that an ancestor-spirit (*saman*), stemming from the blood soul and body soul of an ancestor, waits for an opportunity to reincarnate in a woman of the same blood as himself. The reincarnation of this ancestor is made possible by fertilizing the blood soul (*mogya*) of the wife with the husband's *ntoro* (patriclannish spiritual principle) during intercourse. It can happen that this ancestor-spirit, which is in the soul of the woman's blood, does not like the husband's *ntoro*. He will never accept the fusion of the two bloods nor will he support this detested *ntoro*. The union will, consequently, be sterile. Once the diviners have indicated the cause, the couple has a right to separate, so that each partner can go his own way and procreate (Rattray, op. cit., p. 319). Bailey reports that in case of prolonged sterility the Navaho couples agree to try their luck their own way with a maximum of four partners. This goes to show that infertility is supposed to be related to the relation between the couple and not to the individuals. Nevertheless, if one of the partners is indeed sterile, it is tacitly admitted that it can only be the wife. "If they find one who has children for them, they will live together. If not, *one of the men will stay*

with the woman anyway, maybe" (op. cit. p. 21). We have seen that among
the Samo, sterility is also regarded as a purely feminine affair, the men
always having children one way or another.

All this poses problems. Indeed, if we examine the views on procreation, we notice the predominance of those that recognize only the man's
role or allow shared responsibility for the spouses' contributions in the
creation of the embryo, but with the idea of a continuous fabrication by
the man in the mother's uterus thanks to the semen he provides. Similarly, the collective interrogation on the responsibility in a couple's
sterility shows the existence of theories that consider the couple as a unit,
and not as each of the individuals composing it, and that presupposes
an incompatibility of bloods that a priori could be held neutral. However, in all cases it is nevertheless the woman who is considered to be
responsible for or the victim of sterility. There is obviously a kind of
incompatibility, a contradiction between the premises and the conclusion. How can these points of view be reconcilable? Can they be explained, in their duality, by reasons other than the interplay of social
rules that readily allow a man's sterility to be disguised, whereas a
woman's is always flagrant? And what is wrong with and for the sterile
woman?

We have seen that local theories are based on concrete observations,
some of which are extremely trivial: the evidence of a woman's fertile
period between puberty and menopause, the evidence of the necessity
of sexual relations, but also of their insufficiency. Others, on the contrary,
are all in all more sophisticated: the common nature of sperm and blood,
or at least the fact that sperm has features that allow it to convey several
heritages from one individual to another, the period of adolescent infertility (limited fertility), or the idea of incompatibility of bloods while both
partners can be fertile in other unions. These obvious facts and observations are the basis for theories on respective contributions, the development of the foetus, its nourishment, its transformations, on the ideal
moment to conceive and even on determining the sex of a child. But none
of these theories explains what really happens during the act of procreation. By definition, the mechanism of ovulation is not known, neither is
the existence of spermatozoids. After it thickens due to age, semen is thus
supposed to be the same in all men. There is only the proof that menstruation ceases when the woman is pregnant, which brings us back to
the idea of the woman's responsibility. But what then is the nature of this
infirmity?

= It is not seen as a physiological phenomenon, even when a constitutive organic deficiency is very flagrant, as in the case of total amenhorrhea. Absence of menses always implies an incapacity to conceive. Indeed, a girl who has not reached puberty, a menopausal woman, or a nursing mother who does not menstruate, are not usually fertilizable. Therefore, a woman who has never menstruated is the sterile woman *par excellence*. But no theory considers this state as an explanation on its own. It is at the very most the symptom of something else, which is characterized as an emaciation, a gradual languishing, for which an explanation is warranted. We have seen that the Samo do not bury an adult woman who has never menstruated like they do others. First her kidneys are pierced to let her blood flow ("having one's kidneys crushed" is, moreover, a euphemism for menstruating). The Bobo treat these women when they are dead in the same way as "pariahs", members by birth or sexual contact of groups characterized by the socially defined mark of deviant sexual behaviour, zoophiles, necrophiles, etc., are treated elsewhere in Western Africa. They are not buried but left to rot in the open air in trees or dumped into big rivers. The Bobo woman who has not menstruated is partially and symbolically treated in the same way. The little fingers and little toes are removed from her corpse and thrown in the river as a sign of her sexual deviance.[26]

Conversely, continual menstruation, lasting or prolonged haemorrhages after puberty, also indicate an incapacity to conceive for women whose blood "clots", prefigurements of the embryo, "turn", refuse to coagulate and to "set" and liquefy.

In my opinion these are the effects, non-contradictory in principle, even if they are so in their effects (drying-out, haemorrhages, or their dysentery equivalent), of an infringement of a fundamental rule, that of the order governing the continuity of generations and the functions attributed to each one. The right to sexual intercourse and reproduction is appropriated by a sexually active generation which kept the monopoly of it for themselves. According to Meyer Fortes's expression regarding the first born's special status in the world, everything happens as if there were "a limited fund of male vitality and female fertility", a restricted capital of procreative forces whose management can pass to one generation only to the detriment of the previous one.[27] The vitality of the son comes from the decline of the father's vitality, the fertility of the daughter from the decline of the mother's fertility. It is not possible to mingle the generations in this role without approval for the transfer, nor is it possible to let the upcoming generation enter without a minimum of precautions into the roles and functions of the outgoing generation, or to allow the outgoing generation to make a monopoly of its rights. Everything must be done so that neither party present "oversteps" the other, or "cuts off its path", or "crosses" or "strides" across it, "jumps the queue" or "steals the other's part", all metaphors used in ethnographical reports. A daughter needs the consent of her parents and ancestors before becoming sexually active and again before conceiving. In general, she will not have the right to have sexual intercourse before the rituals and ceremonies either of puberty or of marriage (depending on the society) have been performed. Their aim is to give her adult status and responsibility for her own life. The puberty rituals are carried out, often explicitly, to correctly regulate the flows of menstrual blood, by techniques considered appropriate, such as tying the joints from where the blood is thought to come, fasting, removing objects that are too cold or too wet, intensive heating on beds of hot stones, so that the girl is able to conceive and to obtain the ancestors' consent for this change of role and status. During the puberty sacrifice that her father makes for her, and which never takes place in the rainy season, for fear that the sky's humidity allied to her own prevents her flow of blood from ceasing, the Samo girl, and this time not metaphorically, steps over the ashes of a fire, a loincloth brought by her own mother and the dead body of the sacrificed dog three times, before going to her maternal uncles without looking back. This succession of acts signifies that she officially has the right to encroach upon the functions which until then were her mother's.

Before puberty, children are rarely considered as complete persons. They are not buried in the cemeteries for adults, they are not entitled to a funeral, for this would be treating them as adults who had gone through the normal course of life and in doing so their parents would be pushed beyond that stage. It is, therefore, logical that a mistake of this kind among the Ashanti should entail subsequent sterility for the mother (Rattray, op. cit., p. 61), in principle analogous to future menopause. Whether they are regarded as neutral and defenceless beings (Ashanti) or as being constantly in mortal danger,[28] they are said to be "hot", a metaphor which translates exactly the Samo term to describe their situation. Inversely, having sexual intercourse before puberty is regarding oneself as an adult and assuming the related prerogatives illegitimately and prematurely. Total amenorrhea or absolute sterility, final drying-out of vital fluids, is regarded as a possible sanction for this mistake. Sexual intercourse with little girls before puberty can also entail emaciation and impotence, or the drying-out of the vitality of the male adult partner. This is the case among the Bobo, for instance. What is supposed to be the mechanism of this drying-out? It seems to refer to a general pattern which makes man, producer of sperm, and thus of blood, all through his life, a warm being by nature, contrary to the woman whose nature is to be cold, because she loses her blood and that which comes from the man. Nevertheless, the woman has spells of intense heat when she does not menstruate: childhood, pregnancy, nursing, menopause. Sexual intercourse during these different periods necessarily has to be regulated, because it produces an accumulation of heat. During childhood this accumulation leads to the vital fluids drying out and in the end to sterility. During menopause, it creates excess strength, which is dangerous for others.

Thus, a young Samo woman needs her father's consent to have sexual intercourse. After the puberty sacrifice that he makes for her, she receives the pre-marital lover of her choice at home. But if afterwards it turned out that she was barren, one of the logical explanations put forward would be that she had anticipated the exercise of her right. The Ojibwa also believe that one of the reasons why a woman is sterile is that she must have had sexual intercourse before puberty.[29] For the Ashanti, it was a crime which used to be punished by death or expulsion, and even in 1950 still required a purification sacrifice on the ancestral altar, whereas pre-marital pregnancies after the puberty ceremony were tolerated.[30] So it is truly an offence to the ancestors and an infringement of the social rule that regulates the harmonious and unmuddled succession of generations. Breaking that rule is punishable either socially, death, expulsion, various penalties, or mystically, permanent or temporary drying-out, and hence by the removal of reproduction, for having wrongfully, i.e., without having obtained the right and not at the proper time, "cut off the path" of the previous generation. Similarly, among the Muria, where marriage gives the right to procreate, one of the hypotheses explaining a couple's sterility is that the husband dried up his semen by having made his partner at the *ghotul* pregnant, contrary to the rules (Elwin, p. 291). Be it puberty or marriage, there are social thresholds marked by rites which do not necessarily accompany the event and prior to which sexual relations or conception are not valid, in that they represent too exorbitant an infringement on the exclusive rights of the previous generation which alone consents to its gradual dispossession by appropriate rituals and a mystical approval.

Inversely, it is the young girl's right to have her parents perform the rituals that allow her to accede to sex life, marriage and procreation at the proper time. Not to carry out the operations required for the girl to enter into the generation fit to procreate, at the right time, would be to enviously and selfishly reserve this right to themselves. They would thus encroach upon the girl's rights and condemn her to sterility by an incessant waste of her blood. She is then supposed to "rot" on her feet, because her blood never dries up. "Rotten" or "dried-up" fertility, the result is the same: it is the incapacity to bear fruit.

Among the Nyakusa, a girl is often given to her husband's family long before puberty so that she has time to grow accustomed to him, and incomplete sexual relations (*inter crura*) between them are tolerated.[31] Fathers have the right to prohibit complete sexual intercourse even when their daughters are close to puberty, because as long as the puberty rituals, which are mingled with those of marriage, have not been performed, the young girls are considered to be lent out only. These rituals are long and complex. For the point that concerns us, from the very onset of menstruation and before anything whatsoever is consummated, the girl's female relatives or her mother-in-law make her take several strong and dangerous medicines which symbolize the sexual act and represent the blood of the lineage into which she will enter by marriage. The special plant substances of which the medicines are made are supposed to be the typical supports of the blood of every lineage. In taking them, the young woman comes in contact with a foreign and new blood which will shortly be hers: she mithradatizes herself. This preparation is what will make intercourse with her husband possible. We quote the very words of Monica Wilson's informants: "If we do not give her the *ikipiki* medicine, the blood never *dries up*, and it is the same with *undumila*. If it is not given, she constantly has periods and is barren. Yes, some have a period twice in one month, those who have *rotted*. The *undumila* is given to the girl at once as she grows up (i.e., from the first menstruation), so that she can go about without fear; otherwise, if she *washes* without having had it, then a *heavy* one may walk over her footprints, that is *overstep* her, and she will not bear a child, she menstruates continually.... If the heavy ones have overstepped her, her body *rots* (p. 102; emphasis added).

Between the first appearance of menstruation and the end of the puberty ceremony, the young girl must not be in contact with water. She is not allowed to wash herself for a whole month, or to cross a river (p. 107, p. 125), because that would make her run the risk of rotting, of having heavy periods, in other words, this effect is the same as that of the puberty rituals carried out in the rainy season among the Samo. These are the first references to the association of phenomena that are characterized as wetness and cold and that appear in different spheres: the biological body and the natural world, and that meet at the same time and whose association produces a negative, cumulative effect, an excess in only one of the two registers. This metaphor of excesses, excess of heat that dries out the growing humours of girls before puberty, due to the sexual relations that she had too early and without the father's authorization, excess of humidity that rots the humours of girls whose rituals giving access to sexuality were not carried out at the proper time, is accompanied by that of the transfers between opposing categories. In the Nyakusa symbology, dense, heavy, is opposed to and prejudices empty and light. Meeting a person who is dense and heavy is prejudicial to those who are not and empties them even more of their substance by this contact through haemorrhages or diarrhoea. It is not without interest to note that those who are dense and heavy are sexually active women who have regular and frequent intercourse with their husbands and, by contagion, these husbands themselves. ("Those who are with their husbands are heavy, they are strong... See, the man ejects semen! Does it go inside? The woman becomes heavy and oversteps the bride." p. 102) The people from whom a young girl menstruating for the first time must chiefly be protected are, therefore, her mother and father. As soon as the event is announced, the parents must cease all sexual relations and may not take them up again until their daughter has started to have regular intercourse with her husband after the puberty rituals and has thus in turn become heavy and capable of resisting the negative influence of other heavy people. If the mother continued to have sexual relations at that moment, she would outrageously overstep her daughter's rights, and because of her very density trigger incessant flows of blood in her daughter and condemn her to sterility, for having manifested by her behaviour the will to preserve the exclusive enjoyment of sexual rights within her generation.

The young girl, who is withdrawn during her puberty and marriage ceremonies, is not allowed to see her father, whose sexual power engendered her and whose eclipsing enables her to be a woman (her father makes her put on a robe after the ritual bath: "Dressing her in it means her father has made her grow up. It means: now she is a woman, let her act like a woman.... When you go to your husband it will not be painful. Have intercourse", p. 108). The tacit authorization of the father, who recognizes his daughter as an adult and allows her to accede to sexual life, is also asked of the paternal ancestors of the lineage. They are all present in her, in her blood, and they are kindly asked to retreat, to stand back a little, to leave some free space to the husband's blood, so that the young woman can conceive and bear a child of her husband (p. 112). The ancestors must give up their place and retreat. Sometimes they do not accept it, if they are angry with their descendants for having omitted part of the ritual in their honour. They "attach" the girl's fertility by drying her out. The blood incompatibilities that we mentioned before, namely among the Ashanti and the Samo, are similar explanations: the ancestors refuse to retreat or to bear another blood.

We have seen that when a Nyakusa girl reaches puberty, her parents do not approach each other as long as the girl herself has not slept with her husband. Afterwards the parents may take up their relations again, but they have to practise *coitus interruptus* because the mother must not become pregnant before her daughter. Only then may the parents continue procreating. "If we do that before our daughter, she will never have children and someone could ask us: how can you overstep your daughter like that?" said a Nyakusa informant (pp. 123, 125). Even more Draconian, because there is no compromise possible allowing two generations to exercise the same rights, a mother and her son, or rather a woman and her daughter-in-law cannot have children at the same time. If a woman is pregnant after her son has married a young woman, it is thought that she will fall ill and that her husband will be cursed "for having consented to the marriage of his son with a grown-up woman while the mother was not old yet and had therefore not finished her career."[32] Conversely, if the son has taken away a girl without her father's consent, or has married a grown-up girl when the father consented only to an engagement to a young girl, it is the son and the daughter-in-law who will be sterile. It is said in *Rituals of Kinship among the Nyakusa* that if the mother becomes pregnant after the marriage of the son, at the same time as her daughter-in-law, she makes the subsequent fertility of her children rot by this act ("the fertility of the son and his wife rots", p. 137). In all the cases, it is very clear that between mother and daughter-in-law, that is to say, between people living in the same house, the right to procreate is not to be exercised simultaneously by two successive generations. In short, among the Nyakusa, a girl needs her father's consent to copulate and her mother's consent to conceive.

Even if the disastrous consequences for either generation are not always clear and explicit, the central idea of a capital of vital force which can be held and managed by a single generation only, is widespread, even if it is often covered by a veil of morality. Firth writes that in Tikopia a married son would be ashamed in the presence of people if his mother was pregnant. He adds: "the central idea is that the external evidences of sexual behaviour should not be present in both generations at the same time."[33] In China (Yunnan), it is also shameful for a woman to be pregnant again once a daughter-in-law is brought into the family.[34] The author, Francis Hsu, stipulates that "the function of perpetuating the ancestral line is vested in the father as long as the son is not married, but afterwards it passes to the son." Also, after the marriage of the first son and in any case after the birth of the first grandchild, the parents of the young couple even permanently cease sharing the same room.

So, it is not appropriate to mingle the generations. But, except for the necessary consent of the ancestors and parents to the exercise of sexuality by their children and, thus, to sharing or dispossession of the rights which until then were theirs exclusively, the husbands of the girls must, more generally, by a shift in thinking, overcome something that is seen in collective representation schemas as a natural malevolence of femininity towards the transmission of life. As sovereign distributors of life, women have all the power to refuse it. To the implicit idea that the mother of the bride must consent for her daughter to conceive, to the similar idea of the daughter's dependence on the mother, of their identity, the idea must be added of the daughter refusing to submit herself to her destiny, so there is, consequently, a natural hostility of femininity towards the transmission of life, a hostility which should be overcome by appropriate ritual and social techniques. This fear is expressed often and mainly, but not only, in strong patrilineal societies, either the acts of malevolence or sorcery by the mother-in-law or the bride so that the latter does not bear children are feared, or it is necessary to win the favour mystically of the generative forces typical of femininity. So, among the Azande (Evans-Pritchard, op. cit., p. 402), the hostility of the bride's mother is supposedly accompanied by practices that control the young woman's fertility. Some of her clothing with stains of menstrual blood and nail clippings are hidden in an anthill or in the trunk of a hollow tree. The husband can, so it seems, use the same methods for revenge after having sent back his spouse if he has become aware of these harmful manoeuvres and if the intervention required of his father-in-law has not yielded any result, condemning her in turn to sterility with other men but him. Bailey reports the existence in Navaho matrilineage of several contraceptive plant recipes and practices carried out by the women, such as putting a few drops of menstrual blood or afterbirth in the current of a river (op. cit., pp. 11-12), which does not have the effect here of increasing the menstrual flows, but of reducing them. Adding same to same supposedly suppresses something by reflux, instead of increasing it by osmosis, as was the case among the Nyakusa, but it is the same logical process that is in action. These medicines and practices are indeed aimed at suppressing menstruation, by reflux in the body (p. 25: "it stops the woman from menstruating and sometimes after that, she gets sick from too much blood in her.... Then she takes another medicine to clean this blood out.") We have seen earlier on that in this society, the children stem from the man's blood, but only if it is "stronger" than that of the wife. If it is weaker and cannot assert itself, she will not have children. This shows how little femininity is disposed towards reproduction. The relationship between the two bloods is an antagonistic one. Some "medicines" are supposedly brewed by the mother for the daughters when they first menstruate to strengthen their bloods and for ever prevent them from becoming pregnant. ("If a girl's mother doesn't want her to have a baby, they give her this medicine at her first menstruation. My mother gave it to my half-sister and she has never had any children." p. 26) As for the patrilineal Samo, they believe that a woman has children only in so far as her spiritual components (her individual destiny) wants it. That destiny is itself dependent on her mother's. After the marriage, the son-in-law must, by means of sacrifices, attract the favour of the generative forces that come from his mother-in-law's uterine lineage that are transported by plants soaking in water. Drinking of that same water is what will make his spouse fertile, provided that her individual destiny does not completely prohibit conceiving and that the bloods coming from their ancestors are not incompatible. Sometimes it has no effect. The young woman will then drink the sacrificial generative water from her mother-in-law's lineage. But whether the young bride's fertility stems from the one or the other, it is always the female mystic forces that must be appeased and made favourable to reproduction (Heritier, "L'identite samo", pp. 61-62).

The fathers' consent, the mothers' consent, that of the female principle, and the ancestors' consent reflect the need to respect a fundamental rule: life is to be transmitted according to the normal order of generations. Fear of female sterility, however, reflects the obsession of not being able to do so, because it is always possible to rouse the bad will of one or other of these instances towards oneself or someone else. Because it is not enough to ensure that the respective roles of the successive generations are not confounded, one may not intermingle what should not be intermingled, or cross without precaution: to cross, to mingle blood by marriage or sexual union is a delicate, if not dangerous, affair, and it is not possible either to cross kinds, to make meet what must be separate.

Marriage is a serious affair that concerns adults, because a blood must be found of which the ancestors approve, so that they agree to give up space (Nyakusa) or to tolerate the fusion of their substance with the foreign substance (Ashanti). This explains the importance in this field of the rules of marriage that allow for choices that make up as much as possible for fate and the risks of harmful encounters. Because the penalty for bringing together two incompatible bloods, not accepted by the ancestors, will be a sterile union or the premature death of offspring. However, these unwanted encounters of blood can also come about by other means than by an unfortunate choice of spouse, but produce similar effects. Thus, we have seen the array of precautions surrounding puberty and the first sexual relations of a young Nyakusa girl. Her mother temporarily ceases to have intercourse with her husband so as not to risk "being heavy", attracting to her and confiscating for her benefit the humoral substance and the fertility-to-be of her daughter. The young girl was introduced into the blood of her husband's lineage by taking strong "medicines" (*ikipiki*) that inspire terror. These remedies are ingested with the aim of making the bride a quasi-blood relation of her husband. (Wilson, *Rituals of Kinship*, p. 105): "The medicine... is our kinship, it is our blood... (it) is to create relationship. Using it means that the bride is now of my lineage.") Moreover, they give her strength, because she is empty since her menses, to resist possible contact with "dense" and "heavy" women, who would give her uncontrollable diarrhoea. But, as soon as the girl has copulated with her husband, it is she who becomes dangerous to her own mother, because of the identity of nature that exists between them, because she has mixed her blood with that of another lineage. She must bring her mother symbolically into contact with the blood, foreign to her, as is that of her son-in-law, otherwise it is the mother who will suffer from uncontrollable diarrhoea and will not be able to conceive again. Her daughter would then have overstepped her unduly. To put these different bloods in contact without any risk, the young bride brings her mother a chicken and ears of millet that she rubbed with her hands, with which she has just wiped her husband's genitals after having had intercourse with him (p. 100). She comes in the morning, so that it can be eaten by both her parents if she is the first-born girl (point of inflexion of the new generation), or otherwise by her mother alone. By this symbolic consumption of the son-in-law's body, the parents become like herself one flesh with her husband. Their bloods become mutually tolerant. She says to her mother: "Mother, I have wiped the penis of my husband, I have grown up." (p. 115) With these words and by carrying out the communal ritual, her mother will not have diarrhoea, a discharge by which the organism tries to rid itself of a foreign body (p. 129).

Adultery produces the same effects on the husband, because the "blood" of two men meet in the same matrix. The husband's legs will be swollen, because his vital substance flows back in him, and he will have diarrhoea, a way to evacuate the deleterious contact (p. 132). The danger stems precisely from the encounter with the semen, and thus the blood, of the other man, and not from adultery itself. The husband does not suffer from anything (except jealousy perhaps) if the lover takes care to practice *coitus interruptus* (p. 134). Among the Lovedu, a man cannot "mix" his wives, go from one to another without precaution, without following the rules: he would undoubtedly mix their bloods. And a woman who is made pregnant by her lover is supposedly a serious threat to her husband's health (Krige, op. cit., p. 158).

As we have mentioned before, it is just as impossible to cross kinds as it is to mix bloods and generations with impunity. What does that mean? Every society has its own ideas about what concerns human beings and what does not. It builds an order of things within which social life is lived. Anything that deviates, or short-circuits or contaminates kinds that must be kept separate is dangerous for the individual and for the community. This limited order of things has "short-fallings": incest, homosexuality, onanism; and "beyonds": the sub-real world of divinities and spirits, the extra-human sub-real world of animality and inanimate objects. All the contacts that take place with the outside, with short-fallings and beyonds can themselves be bearers only of sterility, since they deviate from this limited order of things where the social rule that makes the mankind that reproduces and recognizes itself, like to itself, generation after generation.

Sterility, malformation, corruption are the effects of relations with the beneath. The Navaho believe that masturbation among women in early times gave rise to the birth of monsters (Bailey, op. cit., p. 19). As for the Ojibwa, they explain hydrocephaly among young babies born to two married women, an aunt and a niece, as being the result of supposed homosexual relations between them prior to their marriages.[35] The two children are swollen with excess water resulting from these cold and humid relations. Incest, however, is frequently suspected as the main cause of a couple's sterility, because it warms, it dries out or it rots. Many examples are known of this in Africa.

An inventory of what can be found on this subject by gleaning among anthropological literature shows that relations with the beyonds, such as coming in contact with the sacred world, has sterilizing effects too. When a chief is appointed among the Akan, he is hung three times above the black stone of the consecration altar. His body must not come into contact with this altar, because the slightest touch "would weaken his reproductive organs for ever", i.e., he would become impotent, because the consecration altar is a "living force" whose substance is too strong for a human being to bear.[36] Among the Lovedu, when things are not going too well in the country, when there is a drought, all the fires are extinguished with *mufugo*, a special medicine that the queen keeps. Only girls who have not yet reached puberty fetch water for its preparation, and young boys, who have not reached puberty either, carry it carefully to the different villages where a few drops are sprinkled on the fires to extinguish them. Only the old menopausal women may then rake the ashes. For all the others, that is to say, for all the individuals who have reached puberty and can procreate, any contact whatsoever would entail permanent sterility. "It is considered extremely dangerous, liable to rob men and women of their fertility, and great care is thus necessary when working with it." (Krige, op. cit., p. 276) We have seen before that dreaming of intimate contact with evil spirits, diabolical forces, explains the sterility of Ojibwa women who, moreover, become "fatal sorceresses" (Landes, op. cit., p. 37).

We have found only one explicit example of relations with the extra-human sub-real world of the dead, but it is very relevant. The Ashanti believe that female sterility and male impotence are certain to occur when one has dreamed of having sexual intercourse with a dead person who was one's partner when alive (Rattray, op. cit., p. 193). Any widow is also at great risk: she must remain by her husband's body for a couple of days. If his spirit comes back before he finally leaves and in her dreams copulates with her, then she will be irremediably sterile (p. 191).

Animals and the natural world are not dangerous in themselves, if they are properly and sensibly handled, man making use of nature and feeding himself on it. But they become dangerous if they metaphorically overstep man, especially by devouring or holding that very peculiar part of the human body that detaches itself from the woman and the child, that was living flesh and becomes merely dead flesh: the placenta. Giving the placenta to dogs, as the Yanhan do,[37] or to badgers, as the Navaho do (Bailey, op. cit., p. 26), or more generally letting animals devour it, as the Havasupai do (Spier, op. cit., p. 300), putting the afterbirth in the river and letting it swell up, are all acts that entail sterility in women, just like eating the animal-totem of the husband.[38] It is uniting kinds that should normally be kept separate or that should not be joined in that way.

Sterility, a female affair as the objective evidence of apparent biological facts want us to believe, is thus seen mainly as a social sanction within the body, for actions that infringe the law, deviate from the norm, and go beyond limits that are always narrowly defined. Three main faults of behaviour are punished this way: mixing generations, mixing bloods and mixing kinds, when it is done improperly and brutally. But rather than sanction, which implies above all a penalty, it would be better to speak of consequence, of immediate transcription. This direct result can affect the one who breaks the law, or another, or a group. It can also affect in completely different areas which we did not take up here. Acts of transgression of a same order have climatological, meteorological effects via a sort of direct metaphorical transfer from one field to another. Nevertheless, it is always a matter of giving a meaning to, and, above all, of compensating breaches in the order, the balance of the world. These three fields, the biological environment, the social environment and the natural environment (meteorological or other), are regarded as closely connected, because from the sensitive qualities of things man has always constructed systems of interpretation that express at the same time his need to "organize social relations, to forge a system of moral conduct and to solve the problem of man's position in nature," as S.J. Tambiah wrote in 1969.[39]

NOTES

1. Starobinski, Jean, "Sur la chlorose", *Romantisme, Revue de la Société des Etudes Romantiques*, XI, 3, 1981, pp. 113-130 (special issue: Sangs).
2. Durkheim, Emile, *Les formes élémentaires de la vie religieuse*, 6th edition, Paris, PUF, 1979, p. 627.
3. Elwin, Verrier, *The Muria and their Ghotul*, Bombay, 1947.
4. Ashley-Montague, M.F., "Adolescent sterility", *Quarterly Review of Biology*, XIV, 1939, pp.13-34, 192-219.
5. Malinowski, Bronislaw, *The Sexual Life of Savages in Northwestern Melanesia*, London, G. Routledge, 1932, p. 168.
6. Barton, R.F., *Philippine Pagans*, London, G. Routledge, 1938.
7. Rentoul, A.C., "Physiological paternity and the Trobrianders", *Man*, XXXI, 1931, p. 153.
8. Himes, N.E., *Medical History of Contraception*, London, 1936.
9. Pitt-Rivers, G.H.L., *The Clash of Culture and the Contact of Races*, London, G. Routledge, 1927, quoted by Elwin, op. cit., p. 303.
10. Seligman, C.G., *The Melanesians of British New Guinea*, Cambridge, 1910, p. 500.
11. Evans-Pritchard, E.E., "Heredity and gestation, as the Azande see them", *Sociologus*, VIII, 1932, pp. 400-414.
12. Krige, E.J., and Krige, J.D., *The Realm of a Rain Queen*, Oxford University Press, 1943.
13. Junod, Henri A., *The Life of a South-African Tribe*, 2 vol, London, Mac Millan, 1927.
14. Landes, Ruth, *The Ojibwa Woman*, New York, Columbia University Press, 1938, p. 101.

15. Rattray, Robert S., *Religion and Art in Ashanti*, Oford, Clarendon Press, 1927, p. 67.
16. Héritier, F., "Fécondité et stérilité. La traduction de ces notions dans le champs idéologique au stade préscientifique", in *Le Fait féminin*, Paris, Fayard, 1978, pp. 387-396.
17. Lorimer, F., *Culture and Human Fertility. A Study of the Relation of Cultural Condition to Fertility in Non-industrial and Transitional Societies*, Paris, UNESCO, 1954.
18. Christensen, J.B., *Double Descent Among the Fanti*, (Ph. D., Northwestern University, 1952), p. 63.
19. Cf., also the article quoted by Françoise Héritier, "L'identité samo", in *L'Identité*, Paris, Grasset, 1977.
20. Richards, A.I. and Reining, P., "Report on fertility surveys in Buganda and Buhaya, 1952" in F. Lorimer ed., *op.cit.*
21. Héritier, 1978, art. quoted, p.391.
22. Krige, E.J. and Krige, J.D., op. cit., p. 212.
23. Bailey, Flora L., *Some Sex Beliefs and Practices in a Navaho Community. With Comparative Material from other Navaho Area*, Cambridge, Mass., Harvard University, Peabody Museum of American Archeology and Ethnology, Papers, vol. 40, 1950, p. 26.
24. The Ojibwa do not believe that a single act of intercourse can lead to conception, they hold that a man can be the father only if he has had regular intercourse with the mother during four of five months; cf. Dunning, R.W., *Social and Economic Change among the Northern Ojibwa*, Toronto, University of Toronto Press, 1959, p. 147.
25. The Havasupai think that man works constantly to shape what was at the beginning a mere concentration of blood; cf. Spier, L., "Havasupai ethnography", *Anthropological Papers of the American Museum of Natural History*, New York, vol. 24, 1928, p. 116.
26. Héritier, F., "Le charivari, la mort et la pluie", in J. Le Goff and J.C. Schmitt eds., *Le Charivari*, Paris, E.H.E.S.S., Mouton, 1982, p. 357.
27. Cf. Fortes, M., "The first born", *Journal of Child Psychology and Psychiatrics*, XV, 1974.
28. Cf. Héritier, F., in "L'identité samo", art. quoted, p. 57.
29. Hilger, M.I., *Chippewa Child Life and its Cultural Background*, Washington, Smithsonian Institution, 1951, (Bureau of American Ethnology, Bulletin no 146), p. 3.
30. Fortes wrote in 1950 ("Kinship and marriage among the Ashanti", in A.R. Ratcliffe-Brown and D. Forde eds., *African Systems of Kinship and Marriage*, Oxford University Press, 1950): "It is a sin and a crime, for which both parties are nowadays liable to a heavy fine and to public obloquy, for a girl to conceive before her puberty ceremony." And based on Rattray, he added in a note: "Part of the fine is used to procure sheep for a purification sacrifice to the community ancestral stool..."
31. Wilson, M., *Rituals of Kinship among the Nyakusa*, Oxford, University Press, 1957, p. 86.

32. Wilson, M., *Good Company. A Study of Nyakusa Age-Villages*, Oxford University Press, 1951, p. 108.
33. Firth, R., *We, the Tikopia. A Sociological Study of Kinship in Primitive Polynesia*, London, George Allen and Unwin, 1936, p. 492.
34. Hsu, Francis L.K., *Under the Ancestor's Shadow*, New York, Columbia University Press, 1948, p. 110.
35. Landes, Ruth, *Ojibwa Sociology*, New York, Columbia University Press, 1938, p. 53.
36. Danquah, J.B., *Gold Coast. Akan Laws and Customs and the Akim Abuaka Constitution*, London, G. Routledge, 1928, p. 114.
37. Gusinde, M., *Die Feerland-Indianer*, vol. II, *Die Yamana. Vom Leben und Denken der Wassernomaden am Kap Horn*, Vienna, Anthropos, 1937, p. 502.
38. Lagae, C.R., *Les Azande ou Niam-Niam. L'organisation zande, croyances religieuses et magiques, coutumes familiales*, Brussels, Vromant, 1926, (Bibliotheque Congo, vol. VIII), p. 41.
39. Cf. Tambia, S.J., "Animals are good to think and good to prohibit", *Ethnology*, VIII, 1969, p. 459.

Chapter 4

HISTORY OF DISEASES, HISTORY AND DISEASE: AFRICA

E. M'Bokolo

It may seem surprising that diseases, as a subject-matter for study, have until now sparked so little interest among historians of tropical Africa, considering the many connections that can be supposed to exist between morbidity rates and other traditional subjects of Africanist research, such as migration, trade, contacts with the outside, and underpopulation. Indeed, disregarding the studies (a systematic survey of which has yet to be done) written by colonial administrators, doctors and missionaries and containing information and hypotheses about the history of one or several diseases in a specific region,[1] historical research as such began in this field at a very late date. The first noteworthy efforts appeared only in the late 1960s, and were continued by the fairly sparse research of the following decade, in particular the works of S.M. Cissoko, J. Ford, C. Wondji, K.D. Patterson and G. Hartwig.[2]

It was then that people began to recognize the importance and the multiple implications of certain epidemics, the link between large disasters, famine, floods, war, and disease, and the many insights which the study of diseases could offer into the structure and evolution of societies. Part of the reason why these facts were recognized so late, and so hesitantly, was that the researcher would presumably have to possess technical knowledge in biology, ecology, and especially medicine, to undertake historical research on diseases. Moreover, this new field did not seem as glamorous nor as open to polemics as the history of pre-colonial states, African resistance to colonialism, or the conditions leading to underdevelopment, all preeminent topics of research. Finally, the research techniques and the approach developed in the 1960s and 70s for other areas of African history did not seem as operative nor as effective for the history of diseases.

Rather than study a disease or series of diseases in a given region over a specific period, we decided to undertake an overview of current and projected work in this field, with the aim of bringing out a certain number of lines of study. However, as regards the time-frame, we will place the accent on the long 19th century period from 1800 to 1890, and the pivotal period between 1890 and 1930, which marks the beginnings of the subsequent colonialism. There are three main reasons for this choice. Firstly, source materials, which pose a difficult problem (discussed below) are more readily available for this period than for earlier ones. Therefore this period, one of rapid and major transformations in the economy and in political systems, seems to lend itself best to studies which, more than being merely a history of diseases, also attempt to situate them in history. Lastly, problems of interpretation arise even before any great number of concrete studies are available. Accepted ideas are particularly tenacious in this field. A digest of these can be found in a healthily provocative work which purports to make a general appraisal of colonialism in tropical Africa.[3] According to the two authors, it was only with colonialism, and very early on, at the beginning of the 20th century, that effective medical care was introduced, that the major endemic and epidemic diseases began to recede slowly but surely, and that plans were laid to organize decent sanitary conditions. Consequently, "before colonization", the situation in general was one of widespread unhealthiness and permanent morbidity: "a large number of people were ... chronically ill from the time that they were born to the day they died."[4] The African doctors (medicine men) depicted as botanists, priests, detectives, and magicians at one and the same time, in short, as variants of Dr. Faust, had neither any knowledge about diseases nor the means to combat them.[5] It is as though this type of simplistic and manichean interpretation ("before colonization" = negative / "colonization" = positive), very close to the colonial ideology, had found one of its last refuges in the study of diseases after having been expelled from the other branches of African history. What little has been done in this field suggests, however, a much more complex reality, and already justifies fresh interpretations.

For the historian studying one aspect or another of diseases in tropical Africa, one of the peculiarities and difficulties facing him is that he is venturing into a field and intending to take possession of an area previously occupied by other social sciences which have formulated hypotheses, defined issues, or even established research methods from which he may not be able to free himself.

Demographers were the first to examine the effects of diseases on society in Africa. It is true that for a long time most of them merely looked at statistical reports on overall population, and birth and death rates, without referring to morbidity factors or other social facts.[6] The situation changed, however, with the works of R. Kuczynski published between 1939 and 1949.[7] He was the first person to take a two-pronged approach of immediate interest to the historian. The first stage was to sketch a population's historical profile, trace its development, and delineate the main stages of growth and depopulation. He managed to do this despite inaccurate information and, especially, despite the fact that the practice of census-taking began very late, rarely dating from earlier than the First World War. Studying East Africa (Kenya, Uganda, Tanganyika, and Zanzibar) in particular, he strove to refute the widely held view that the population had decreased considerably in the period preceding colonization and then began to grow at the end of the 19th century under the shelter of the colonial pax.[8] Based on the accounts of explorers or travellers who, owing to their education or interests, were especially attentive to demographic features, he suggested that the population prior to 1880 had been greatly underestimated, and that whatever its size and growth trends, it had begun to fall in the 1890s, a trend which continued until about 1920. It is in this first stage, when studying numerical changes in population, that Kuczynski brings in the question of diseases: he attributes the supposed decrease of 1890—1920 to the spreading of diseases (whether old or new), facilitated by the colonial takeover and "the breakdown of tribal life". The second aspect of Kuczynski's approach is to study those demographic factors, such as fertility and above all mortality, that are most affected by disease. From there he is able to trade the origins, routes and degree of prevalence of venereal and major endemic diseases.[9] In the light of this research, many demographers took a closer look at low density areas, which they had previously defined less as areas of high mortality than as areas of low fertility. In Central Africa, where most work of this kind was done, they tried to show that the low density was undoubtedly a long-standing characteristic and that the low fertility was due to the slow spread and eventual entrenchment of venereal diseases.[10]

The questions raised by the demographers weighed heavily in subsequent research in different fields of study, which explains why in an anthropological work on the Bandia of Central Africa, E. de Dampierre studied a demographic trend which, to judge from the reports of the colonial administration and the impressions of those involved, looked like "collective suicide".[11] In the space of half a century, from 1900 to 1960, the rough figures on population show a clear decrease, and this is confirmed by oral information. While internal migration, both forced and voluntary, must be taken into account as part of the explanation, the population's state of health is also incriminated. The people suffered from alcoholism and, above all, endemic diseases (smallpox, sleeping sickness, leprosy), or sterility-causing diseases (gonorrhoea and syphilis). Administrative reports and oral traditions make repeated reference to these diseases, but modern European doctors have instead laid the blame on damaging administrative policies (forced labour, displacement of villages) which, they say, created the perfect conditions for the diseases to spread. Depending on the situation and the point of view adopted, then, disease is seen either as one of the prime causes of depopulation or as a deterioration attributable to other factors. If we than attempt to situate diseases historically, we find that most of them appeared at different times. Oral traditions from the last third of the 19th century allude to smallpox in particular, but all agree that syphilis postdates colonial occupation. Administrative reports, for their part, note the successive appearance of smallpox, sleeping sickness, and leprosy, while malaria and parasitoses seem less linked to any specific set of circumstances. Our questions therefore can and must be put differently to try and establish, in addition to an accurate chronology of these diseases, those factors which caused or contributed to the outbreak, spread or worsening of a given disease in a specified period in history.

G. Sautter took an approach somewhat along these lines in his geography of underpopulation in Equatorial Africa.[12] In general, Africanist geographers adopted demographers' concern with regional differences in population density and the widespread underpopulation in Africa.[13] In Equatorial Africa, several areas of very low density with "many factors of depopulation" have been discovered alongside comparatively well-populated regions. In the first half of the 20th century, those factors were, in particular, emigration, whether voluntary or under constraint, the famine of the 1920s, and high mortality from disease. Information on the causes of death, though often scanty, points to several diseases which struck with marked frequency and severity: this is the case of malaria, trypanosomiasis, leprosy and pulmonary diseases in Woleu-Ntem, a low-density region of Gabon. However, as G. Sautter himself points out, "the difficulty with this nosological picture is to distinguish permanent characteristics, a reflection of the physical and human environment, from features belonging to the specific conditions of the period."[14] Thus, pulmonary ailments can be attributed up to a certain point to the harmful effects of altitude, while leprosy, to judge by the improved techniques for isolating diseases, seems to be of relatively ancient date. The other diseases can be more accurately dated: they are linked to the conditions existing during the early stages of colonization. The ravages of malaria can be explained by the low resistance of bodies weakened by a long succession of food shortages, while sleeping sickness, formerly confined to a small number of households, found in the recently-built trails and in the constant movement of migrant workers the ideal means of settling into new regions and extending its territory.

This brief review of a few key studies will allow us to take stock of the attainments of research into diseases within the social sciences other than history. As a matter of fact, all of them call on the historian, particularly in so far as they illustrate with each case study the pressing need for a thorough and accurate chronology of the different diseases in a region. But a history of diseases has far more ambitious aims than simply drawing up a chronology. In the works mentioned above, diseases slip in by the back door, so to speak, they appear incidentally, marginally, as just one factor among others used to account for what are considered to be more fundamental phenomena. The whole point of a history of diseases, on the contrary, is to focus attention on diseases, to make them the main target of study, to examine them in themselves as collective phenomena which have their own evolution and are liable to have an impact in areas as diverse as demography, economics, customs, etc., or to add their effects to those of other social facts. Such a study, if con-ducted analytically, can take one particular disease and follow it over a relatively long period of time, examining its development and each of its effects. In a synthetical approach, it can also identify specific sets of circumstances in given places, and pinpoint the various diseases whose many inter-connections and links with the society as a whole will then be studied.

These aspirations run up against formidable technical obstacles, how-ever. Historical reflection on diseases, if it is truly to flourish, must be based on chronological, geographical, quantitative, sociological, and other types of data which must be sufficiently accurate, ample and varied. The first thing, then, is to find the facts, that is, formulate questions and elaborate techniques through which the facts can be established. Since the history of Africa has been written in the past few decades thanks to new techniques for gathering, criticizing and inter-preting traditions and other oral information, such oral sources are obviously the first that come to mind for establishing the basic facts about diseases. They have, however, proven to be less fruitful on that count than for political history or economic facts. We must immediately qualify that statement, however, by distinguishing roughly between two types of region. The first type involves regions in which diseases, or more precisely, widespread endemic diseases and epidemic outbreaks affecting the entire social group have been relatively rare, or have been widely spaced in time or not particularly severe. Oral sources remain remarkably silent in these cases. That does not mean, of course, that the population has never been stricken by serious diseases. It is as though, with the disaster past, the group had decided to erase it from collective memory or had found no reason to remember it. This situation is not unique to African history. In studying plague epidemics in Western Europe during the Middle Ages, J.N. Biraben and J. Le Goff similarly noticed "the silence of the written sources". The conclusion they drew is valid for Africa as well as Europe: "Men see only what they understand, and put into writing (we would add: commit to collective memory) only what they feel merits being passed on to posterity."[15] What we are calling into question with these remarks is not oral sources in themselves, but social groups in their capacity for sidestepping or concealing certain facts.[16] Fortunately, there is a second type of region, comprising what might be called areas of recurrent disaster. Here, it is easier for the historian to find facts on diseases. These areas experience a wider range of disasters (famine, drought, epizootics, plagues of locusts, etc.) which strike regularly. While diseases still have a profoundly disturbing effect on the social order and social relations, they seem more familiar than in the first type of region. This is notably the case in the African Sahel, on the edges of the Sahara desert. The oral information, compiled in time and recorded in several "Chronicles", underscores just how frequently disasters occurred, diseases being but one aspect of these, and how much store communities set by remembering them. The works of S.M. Cissoko and M. Tymowski[17] on the bend of the Niger show that the 16th century, a period of economic prosperity under the hegemony of the Songhai emperors, was spared such disasters: we know of only three unidentified, and apparently mild, epidemics. On the other hand, the political disruption and commercial difficulties of the 17th and 18th centuries are directly linked, first as cause and then as effect, to disasters of all kinds: there were thirteen in all, the most serious of them lasting eighteen years (1738—1756), and including seven epidemics of "plague".[18] These problems continued into the 19th century, a period for which M. Tymowski has counted twenty-three disasters in Oualata, fifteen of them epidemics and fourteen in Tichitt, six of which were epidemics, usually of small-pox.[19] While it is relatively easy to establish the number and chronology of these outbreaks, the same is not true for their effects. We can see clearly how economic problems made it easier for diseases to ravage weakened bodies, and how the frequency of epidemics made it difficult to rebuild an economy. But how many people were killed by disease? Most often, we meet with indications such as: "the disease took a great toll", or "God alone knows the exact number." Another question, one that arises for highly hierarchical trading societies, is that of the relationship between mortality and social groups. Oral traditions, written down by the literate members of the groups, take care to give the names of eminent persons who have died, but mention only in passing the great number of deaths among the slaves. Finally, the part that these epidemics played in the formation and transformation of sensibilities is also imperfectly conveyed.

The problems are equally as great, however, as far as written sources are concerned. The number of texts on diseases and health conditions in tropical Africa, almost all of them written by Europeans, grew steadily throughout the 19th century, as the continent became increasingly important for the European countries for trade and, soon afterward, for colonialism. The problems posed by these texts are greater or smaller depending on the type of information they contain.

Some of them, which describe a particular disease at a given time and when they take the form of an unbroken series, may give rise only to an analytical history of the disease in question. Thus, for example, an analytical history of yellow fever in Senegal could be written on the basis of the sparse data from the colonial archives. A fair amount of information exists for the 19th century. The disease, which had stricken a few times before 1800, caused no fewer than eleven deadly epidemics during the 19th century.[20] After two outbreaks for which we have only the dates, 1816 and 1828, it reappeared in 1830 taking "a great toll", in 1837, killing 46 out of 160 Europeans, and in 1859, causing the deaths of 162 Europeans. It returned again in 1866-8, "devastating the natives" before being unleashed in 1878 into "the largest epidemic that has ever stricken Senegal" (51% of the Europeans there died).[21] Other less serious yellow fever epidemics were to break out in 1880, 1881, 1882 and 1900-1. With the chronology established, problems begin to arise when an attempt is made to go beyond that stage. Firstly, it is difficult to map out the area reached by successive epidemic outbreaks. The sources, faithfully reflecting the concerns of colonial administrators, rarely speak of anything but the coast and those few points inland where colonial rule had been established. It might be concluded from this that yellow fever was essentially a coastal disease in the 19th century and erupted in regular epidemics imported from ports neighbouring Senegal.[22] Such a conclusion is, however, debatable. We find that beginning in 1878, when the texts begin to mention the interior, each yellow fever epidemic in Senegal spread to the Sudan by means which are still relatively unknown.[23] A further difficulty lies in discovering the effects of these epidemics on African populations, and in particular, their morbidity and mortality rates among the Africans. All of these texts take a whites-centred view of diseases and their effects. There are plenty of figures for Europeans. Africans appear only between the lines, in vague expressions ("ravages", "a great toll") or by way of comparison with the Europeans. In evaluating these epidemics in 1901, one doctor simply noted that: "Yellow fever, when it erupts in Senegal, does not spare the natives: in 1830, at Goree in the Cape Verde peninsula and in Saint-Louis, it carried off a large number of blacks, in at least the same proportions as the Whites."[24] Thirty years later, the point of view had not changed: "Nor did commentators neglect to note the fate of the natives during epidemics.... The native population is stricken by yellow fever only at the same time that the Europeans themselves fall ill."[25] These comments on yellow fever in Senegal can also be applied to the other diseases which, during the same period, appeared outside Senegal in the other coastal regions occupied by Europeans. That explains, then, why texts purporting to be histories based on such sources as these are by and large merely studies of the difficulty Europeans encountered in entering a new health environment, histories of the life and death of a minority foreign to Africa.[26]

The other category of written sources belongs to the genre of "medical geography", a very prolific genre which includes dozens, perhaps hundreds, of books and articles. There is a striking diversity in the titles among the works on Africa: "medical geography" is one, of course, but there are also "medical topography", "natural history", "medical notes", "considerations on hygiene", "medical round"; we also find more neutral, less eloquent headings ("general" or "practical considerations", "field notes", "observations", "remarks", etc.) which we can nevertheless recognize as belonging to this genre from the author's name and the contents. Published continuously for over a century (from 1825 to about 1930), these texts offer a certain diversity owing to the conditions in which they were written. The first ones, those from the 19th century, look at a specific, more or less extensive region, with the theoretical aspiration of describing and explaining the diseases found in that region, and the practical concern of providing doctors with a guide for their diagnoses, giving governments suggestions on health measures to be taken, and furnishing future colonists with valuable advice to be followed in regions that were considered "the white man's grave".[27] The headings in these books, almost always the same, can be found, for example, in the many works by the Sierra Leonean doctor F.J. Africanus Horton, who seems to best illustrate the African "medical geography" genre for this period.[28] Occasionally with the aid of statistics, he writes on topography, botany, climates and seasons, mortality, the most common diseases, and some medical techniques of the African peoples. Horton endeavours to show that soils, climate and vegetation have a direct impact on health. According to him, there is a direct correlation between physical environment, diseases and behaviour, and races, linked to different environments, have varying nosological profiles. Starting in about 1890, when more conquests and more possession-taking missions were carried out, "medical geographies" tended no longer to describe a localized area, they rather drew a broad outline of "the pathology of the regions travelled by the Army columns."[29] From then on, greater importance is given to enumerating and describing the diseases found in the various regions. At this point, indications, often in statistical form, begin to appear on the spreading of diseases for which satisfactory morbidity indices can be calculated. The authors also point out the local names for the diseases, as well as treatments applied and their efficacity. Sometimes, but only too rarely, the groups were asked to tell how long a given disease had existed among them. Starting in about 1914, localized studies again predominate, but there are a few innovations. "Medical geography" discovers a new area of study, the colonial towns, whose pathology is seen as differing significantly from that of the villages.[30] Moreover, nosographical description decreases while vaccination and prevention campaigns are complacently described.

Despite their relative diversity, these "medical geographies" all raise identical problems. The abundant information they contain is more qualitative than quantitative, and does not readily permit a close study of the effects of diseases. This qualitative information in itself is not easy to interpret, particularly in texts pre-dating 1900. The difficulty stems from the fact that not only do diseases and their effects change, but the very way in which doctors conceive of diseases itself changes. A fruitful use of these sources requires an analysis of all the medical vocabulary and the successive systems of reference adopted in the writings of colonial doctors, which convey more than simply positive knowledge. Finally, many of these texts labour under a rigid conception of the geographical dependency of pathogenic complexes. While a very few authors look to "medical geography" merely for "the causes which can influence states of health",[31] most authors are characterized by a narrow geographical determinism according to which a geographical environment or an ecological profile is permanently and unilaterally linked to a particular disease or cluster of diseases.[32] Such an approach is apt to preclude a fruitful historical use of these texts, even if they have the advantage of suggesting the need for a synthetical and general study of diseases by showing that, within a given place, there are always several diseases, that affects are either compounded or offset by one another, and that the state of health of a given group is not unaffected by the other elements that make up and shape its existence.

It would therefore appear that, despite the reservations expressed above, a history of diseases can delve deep into these sources and can incorporate the issues elaborated previously and outside it by other disciplines. Such a history must assume the task of studying not only epidemic and pandemic diseases, dramatic and massive events which demand a certain amount of attention, but also endemic diseases, common, everyday diseases which nevertheless affect individuals and social groups. Clearly, this history will have to explore along several different pathways: we will only deal here with two major ones where greater efforts are most needed.

The first line of study, derived partially from work in demography and geography, would give priority to the study of diseases as they relate to economics and demography. Epidemiological studies by doctors have in fact demonstrated the existence in a given region, and even more so on a continental scale, of a number of "epidemiological landscapes."[33] This term denotes all of the pathological states of a given population as well as the various kinds of factors underlying them. It is also recognized that in conditions of relative isolation a complex process of adaptation takes place between man and the various pathogenic agents, ending in a delicate balance between the population group and diseases, with the former acquiring a certain number of immunities, since it is in the interests of parasites and other viruses, if they are to survive, not to kill all their hosts. These epidemiological landscapes obviously reflect the geographical environment and, insofar as the geographical environment must be distinguished from the human environment, all of the population group's activities, its relations with its environment, and its organization. We can see that "medical geography" has much to contribute to such a study. Furthermore, from another point of view, the state of a population group, its density, but also its growth curve and productivity, is an excellent indicator of pathological conditions. Knowing that none of these epidemiological landscapes is immutable, the historian tries both to reconstruct the successive landscapes in a given place and to determine the different factors, the various situations which obtained at the time of the changeover or which can shed some light on it.

By all indications it will doubtless be difficult, not to say impossible, in the study of Africa, to map out all of or even the most significant of these epidemiological landscapes, whereas it is easier to perceive factors or situations of abrupt change of slow transition (migration, development of trade, contacts with the outside world), which have furnished African historiography with its major themes.

Since these are more or less lengthy periods of delicate equilibrium between a population group and its diseases, we are, for the time being, reduced to guesswork. What little information historical demography provides is a good point of departure. All of the cases of this kind are in fact similar. There were probably more environments than appears at first glance in which man was lastingly stronger than the pathogenic agents. Sometimes this was the result of the gradual immunization of the population, the development of effective medical and health practices, or good judgment in choosing village sites. An important advance will have been made once a significant survey of these cases has been made. In many instances, this will initially require merely asking new questions of sources that are already known. We will content ourselves here with the example of the historiographically significant Bantu-speaking peoples of South Africa.[34] At first, and for a long time, they were studies from the point of view of political history with the emphasis on the Zulu revolution by Shaka at the beginning of the 19th century that led to the formation of centralized monarchies and nation states. When, much later, attempts were made to explain the revolution, very few scholars suggested that the demographic factor might have been a cause, that population growth was particularly strong in the second half of the 18th century, creating unbearable pressure on the arable land, and thus a sort of land hunger which in turn caused conflicts between neighbouring groups, whence the political revolution. One of its objectives even seems to have been a Malthusian solution to the demographic problem by institutionalizing murderous wars and prolonged mandatory celibacy. Now these relatively high population growth rates precede the XIXth century and were mainly through a deliberate series of choices. The Bantu-speaking peoples came from the north at an unknown date, probably before the XVth century, eventually settled on the highlands, where neither malaria nor tse-tse flies existed, and were afterwards careful to avoid all contact with Europeans. As a consequence, tubercu-

losis, smallpox, syphilis and measles were unknown among them until
the XIX century. The population was maintained because there was a
low mortality rate. Conversely, the forest area of Central Africa seems
to have long been characterized by low density, a high death rate
reflecting unfavourable biological and health conditions, and the en-
demicity of several serious diseases.[35]

As far as the factors of abrupt change and situations of transition are
concerned, they are more numerous, and lend themselves to an easier
formulation of hypotheses. Here again, the situations seem to have been
quite varied. The more or less massive "migrations" covering fairly large
distances that were so numerous in the history of tropical Africa offer
the first example of these times of abrupt change. In some cases, populations from complex environments with a multitude of diseases, but
which had acquired the necessary immunities, settled in regions where
they drastically upset bio-pathological balances without suffering any
harm themselves. This seems to have been the case of the Bantu migrations in Central and Southern Africa.[36] What took place was probably
not so much a massive invasion of warlike peoples as a slow infiltration
of groups with a mastery of agriculture and metalworking who were
inured to the diseases concomitant with deforestation and the growth of
relatively densely populated villages, and who brought with them
pathogenic agents, more than weapons, were what allowed them to
settle despite the presence of indigenous peoples, Pygmies in Central
Africa, and Khoikhoi and San in the south. In other cases, migrant
populations from relatively disease free areas found themselves faced
with diseases in their new environments against which they were unable
to find the proper defences. This occurred with the Kololo, for example,
one of the many groups which fled the Zulu revolution in Southern
Africa. After wandering about for some time they settled in Barotseland
on the upper Zambezi in about 1835. This highland people found that
they had fallen into a trap in these regions, which flooded regularly and
where malaria was endemic. In fact, it was malaria that decimated the
population, contributing to its political disintegration around 1865. The
Kololo were aware of this, and their efforts to regain healthier regions
were foiled by the greed of their neighbours who were after the same
land.[37] Again in the XIX century, the Fang had an equally disastrous
experience in migrating from Cameroon to Gabon, where not only local
endemic diseases but also diseases imported from Europe awaited
them.[38]

Prolonged contacts with the outside world provide the second example of a relatively stable bio-pathological situation being upset. The

history of the exchange of diseases between Africa and the other continents and, in particular, of the introduction by Europeans of various
diseases from Europe and the New World into Africa has yet to be
written. However, profound regional differences are already apparent.
Western Sudan, which was opened up at an early date to trans-Saharan
trade, and the Atlantic coastal regions, which were involved in sea trade
from the 15th century onward, were the first to experience diseases from
abroad. The circumstances and effects of this experience have not yet
been elucidated.[39] But the fact that it happened relatively early undoubtedly explains why, when trade and direct relations between Africa and
the outside world increased sharply around 1830, these areas were the
least affected by diseases from abroad. In contrast, it was precisely in the
XIX century that regions which had hitherto been relatively isolated
underwent the first drastic upheaval of their epidemiological landscapes. Nowhere can the extent and complexity of this upheaval be seen
more clearly than in East Africa.[40]

Evidence that the peoples of this region were relatively isolated prior
to the XIX century can be found in that there seem to have been few
large-scale migrations and trade relations with the outside appear to
have been marginal. The main innovation of the XIX century was the
breaking down of the barriers between peoples following a boom in
trade and the integration of these peoples into a single vast economy
controlled by the state of Zanzibar. Increasing numbers of larger and
larger caravans departed from the coast for the interior in search of ivory
and slaves. Starting around 1860, their activity took them regularly to
the west of Lake Tanganyika, in what is now Zaire. The ivory and slave
trades brought new men, Arabs and Swahili, into the interior from the
coast. But the population movements thus created were more complex
than the mere comings and going of foreign merchants. Here and there
ethnic groups enlisted in the new system of trade and began criss-cross-
ing in their turn the areas most advantageous to trade. Another substantial flow moved from the interior towards the coast, as each year
thousands of slaves reached the plantations of Zanzibar and Arabia.
Parallel to this trade directed from the exterior, a large local and regional
commerce grew up in foodstuffs and crafts.[41] The migration of peoples
from the north (Masai, Somali) or the south (Wangoni) affected many
parts of East Africa. The XIX century therefore appears in the accounts
of travellers, missionaries and doctors, and in some oral traditions that
are difficult to interpret, as a century in which new diseases irrupted and
old diseases, until then localized, spread irresistibly, with venereal diseases, diseases of the digestive tract, smallpox and cholera regularly

erupting into deadly epidemics. Smallpox, which seems to have been introduced into the region during this period, is described by all travellers as "one of the most fatal diseases" and even "the greatest and most terrible plague" among all ethnic groups, though details have yet to be found on the chronology of outbreaks and their statistical impact. More is known about cholera, however.[42]On the coast, it broke out in regular epidemic waves: between 1817 and 1899 there were six epidemics, which were simply local outbreaks of pandemics from the Indian subcontinent, with which East Africa maintained close economic relations. These cholera epidemics probably struck the entire region, as travellers' accounts note their effects in places as far apart as Buganda, Rwanda and the Masai and Galla countries. In some places, these diseases spread independently of contact with foreign traders or of any other factor. Other disasters, in particular drought and famine, thus played a significant role: there were several of these, either localized or widespread (probably in 1830, 1840, 1860 and 1880). Each time, populations fled and regrouped in regions with an abundance of water or food, thus creating the ideal conditions for the transmission of disease to weakened and unimmunized individuals. We can see from this that epidemics must never be studied independently of other disasters.[43] Another factor also helped spread or contain the effects of disease, hygiene, especially when there was a great deal of intermingling among populations as a result of increased migratory flows, the growth of large commercial centres, and the creation of zones of shelter during food shortages or climatic crises. Though the data is incomplete, it appears that disease took a greater toll among Africans than among Arab and Swahili traders, whose Moslem faith imposed relatively strict rules of personal hygiene. The role of these two factors confirms that the history of disease must also cover the study of diet, lifestyle, and hygiene. In the absence of any statistical data, it is difficult to determine the consequences of these disasters on the demographic evolution of East Africa during this period. Moreover, that evolution probably varied from region to region. According to some authors, epidemics, even in combination with other disasters (famines, slave raids, wars) caused only localized depopulation, and there was an overall rise in population. This view is based on various indications, in particular the wider use of more productive and nutritious food crops (rice and maize), the settling and clearing of new land, and disputes over land, interpreted as a sign of heightened demographic pressure.[44] According to others, given the newness and frequency of the diseases, it is impossible that they did not lead to a large decrease in population. The two schools of thought, starting from the new light cast by the history of diseases, interpret differently the highly important fact of the development of slavery throughout the XIX century. For some, the acquisition of slaves who then became part of lineages was an expression of the need to rebuild groups whose numbers were dwindling under the impact of epidemics. Others see it, on the contrary, as the sign of a prosperous economy, of a large population with a constantly growing need for manpower to provide for its subsistence and replace the men engaged in more remunerative activities. The same observations can be made about the development of sorcery. In some areas, there were more accusations of sorcery as new diseases, the greater number of sudden deaths during epidemics, and the abnormally high death rate in general, were put down to the ill will of certain individuals.[46] This theory is attractive, but flawed. Firstly, facts of another kind have been advanced to explain, in those instances where it has been observed, an increase in cases of sorcery (sharper economic and political competition; a feeling of insecurity; the hitherto inexistent possibility of profiting from accusations of sorcery by selling persons convicted of sorcery to slave traders). Secondly, in many regions, references to sorcery did not become more common. Instead, they seem to have given way to new beliefs.[47]

These last remarks lead us to other matters. The historical study of diseases is also concerned with apprehending these disasters in their multiple and complex relations with society as a whole.

With this in mind, we must first study medical practices and knowledge. The historian feels himself much more at a loss in this area than the anthropologist. Thanks to ethnographical monographs and the more recent works of medical anthropology, however, detailed descriptions of the medical systems in many regions of Africa are already available. In a number of cases, these descriptions are little more than simple catalogues, which nevertheless have the advantage of aiming for comprehensiveness, of the local interpretations of particular illnesses or of illness as a principle, that is, as a disorder in an individual or a community, of different healing techniques, and of theories on life and death. In certain cases, however, an attempt has been made to organize these different facts into coherent systems of ideas, interpretations and practices. It is thus felt that, unlike Western societies, which are more concerned with health than with illness, "traditional" African societies are overly preoccupied with illnesses, how to interpret them, and the means of combatting them. Illnesses, because they are omnipresent and a constant challenge to individuals and groups, seem to be one of people's main preoccupations. Medical knowledge is organized into hierarchical levels, hence its peculiarity of being both disseminated within the society (the knowledge of individuals and of heads of family) and maintained exclusively by a specialized group, with each level intervening for a specific illness, or at a particular stage in the progress of an illness as the case may be. Not only do this knowledge and these practices call on positive knowledge about the body, substances for healing or preventing illness, or certain surgical techniques, they also convey an ideology, elements that are not properly speaking scientific. This prompts J.M. Janzen, for one, to remark that: "An important facet of African medicine is the way it aims at erecting a sound moral order, a preventive social construction, rather than at getting rid of particular illnesses as they appear."[48] The concept of illness and all those concepts associated with it are thus not an independent domain. It is not only a biological or mental disorder in an individual, but also all sorts of misfortunes affecting his social position that are considered to be illnesses. Even if a restrictive view of illness is adopted, we find that defining illness and its symptoms goes hand in hand with elucidating its causes: illness can be an act of (the) god(s), which implies not so much divine intervention as an upsetting of the physiological balances; it can also result from the ill-meaning acts of men.[49] But neither of these two etiological categories is rigidly linked to an unchanging group of illnesses: the malevolence of men can cause illnesses which under different circumstances are interpreted as god-sent illnesses, but it also results in misfortunes which, stricto sensu are not illnesses. Another characteristic of these practices is what was recently brought to light as the concept of "medical pluralism",[50] flowing directly from the plurality of systems of interpretation and etiological categories. This is where, within a given society, and during a particular period, there are several therapeutic possibilities, each with its specialist healers, its etiological system and its treatment techniques: each illness gives rise to a choice between the different possibilities. It is at this point in particular that one major element of the therapeutic system comes into play: the group of relatives and next of kin who take charge of the sick person(s), formulate assumptions about the causes of the ailment, and choose the most appropriate therapy, often after a certain amount of trial and error.[51]

Faced with all these materials and assumptions, the historian feels himself somewhat encumbered. It seems difficult to move from anthropology to history. In his history of the Kuba, based on a corpus abundant in oral traditions, Jan Vansina recently demonstrated that it is difficult, if not impossible, to construct a satisfactory history of ideologies, beliefs, conceptions and sensibilities, in short, an "intellectual history", for the period preceding colonization.[52] The particular questions that the historian asks more often than not remain unanswered. We can validly assume that the conceptions, knowledge and practices relating to diseases are old. But just how old are they? To what particular conditions (and what types of conditions, health, demographic, political, religious ...) are they attributable? Do this knowledge and these practices have some characteristics that have been permanent and unchanging and others that have changed more frequently? A number of such questions could be asked, questions which seem to focus on elementary problems of chronology and periodization but which in fact raise the fundamental problem of the emergence, duration, permanence and transformations, whether partial or total, major or minor, of medical and health practices. Here again, however, the sources do not supply enough information to answer these queries. The written sources, viewing medical practices from the outside, provide a good chronological framework, but the information is of uneven quality. Oral sources give no information for before the end of the XIX century. These sources (biographies of old healers, descriptions of medical theories and practices, ethnographic records) are often lacking in chronological depth.

As for the history of diseases themselves, the study of medical knowledge and practices can be carried out analytically or synthetically. The analytical approach examines in particular all of the concepts and practices relating to one particular disease and, in addition to a relatively accurate chronology, provides good insights into the mechanisms by which cultural characteristics spread or are borrowed. The best known example is inoculation against smallpox.[53] This practice came to light through external sources: accounts of slaves imported into North America revealed, in the beginning of the 18th century, that inoculation against smallpox was a well established custom in central and western Sudan, to which it may have been introduced by Arab and Berber traders. Smallpox, whose exact distribution in the early 18th century is not yet fully known, seems nevertheless to have spread subsequently as a result of population migrations and trade, though the practice of inoculation did not follow the same routes. Certain populations adopted it while others, such as the Dahomey, formulated a religious aetiology of smallpox that excluded all preventive practices;[54] elsewhere, inoculation was widely used up to the end of the XIX century, and disappeared completely or became clandestine after health measures were introduced by the colonial authorities, who remained hostile towards the technique.

The synthetical approach, which disregards specific diseases to concentrate on nosological concepts and medical and health practices as a whole, is really feasible and satisfactory for previous epochs only for those regions where sufficiently varied sources are available. This is mainly the case for the coastal regions, as many old accounts of journeys over the years are available, fortunately supplemented by the contributions of oral sources. The historian's methods here closely resemble those of the anthropologist, though the historian's conclusions diverge considerably from the anthropologist's assumptions. Three examples give a fairly good illustration of these differences, which show the need for a greater sharing of ideas. Firstly, there is the distribution of medical knowledge within the society. The studies of medical practices in the Ashanti kingdom in the XIX century suggest that rather than being disseminated within the various levels of society, medical knowledge had become the exclusive speciality of a professional corps of herbalists, surgeons and physicians under the control of a high dignitary, the Nsumankwahene, very close to the king (Asantehene) and known for his medico-pharmacological knowledge.[55] This situation had many implications: the medical corps strove to enrich its body of knowledge, particularly by incorporating foreign knowledge and practices (most often Moslem, but European as well); aetiological conceptions changed rapidly, diseases being interpreted more as biological and physiological disturbances than as the effects of social disturbances; finally, the preoccupation with healing diseases after the event seems to have given way to a wish to prevent them through strict hygiene, the isolation of certain sick persons, and inoculation against smallpox. It was tempting to connect these innovations with the emergence of a strong bureaucratic state, but this was not borne out in the other states existing at the same time. Are we to believe, then, that some particular factors came into play, as for example, disastrous populations trends in the state's central regions or the enormous military needs of political leaders?[56] Another example of the new assumptions being formulated by historians concerns the dominant preoccupations within a society. There is a tendency to question the image of "traditional" societies as being more concerned about diseases than about health. The case of the Ashanti kingdom, discussed above, already suggests a different situation which, furthermore, was changing. The case of the Loango coast tends to establish an even more interesting model of change.[57] It seems that until the 17th century, the ideology and therapeutic institutions connected to the state were concerned above all with the good health of the king and his subjects, and the fertility of the land. This political orientation has been seen as a "mirror image"[58] of the political and economic state of the kingdom, which had until then succeeded in preserving its unity and prosperity. It was only at the end of the 17th century that things began to change, and as the black slave trade boomed, the state crumbled and political power was fragmented, insecurity grew, and venereal diseases made frightening inroads. The main concerns then became control over trade, the acquisition of material possessions, theft, "natural" or intentionally provoked diseases, and the means of healing or guarding against them. Should we draw the general conclusion from this that the dominant preoccupations observed from the end of the last century and which gave priority to disease arose from a prolonged deterioration of general living conditions? Whatever the case may be, these two examples furnish the subject-matter of the third question, which involves the collective orientation of medical practice. Current studies have shown that in most cases the sick person is rarely alone in dealing with his disease or his healers. Now it has been observed that on both counts, throughout the XIX century, the sick person took care of his illness on his own: healing techniques mainly involved products and substances to be used by the individual; even when a disease was interpreted as "a man-sent disease", the result of ill will or an attack, the "healer" was not called in to reconcile the individual with his social environment, but rather to enable him to ward off an attack or turn it back against its author.[59]

These developments have shown, in a certain number of cases, that political leaders and the state played a central role in the various changes in therapeutic systems. One wonders if it is possible to draw a few specific correlations between political structure and political practice on one hand, and the field of disease and medical and health practices on the other. This question is neither new, nor is it specific to the African region. Virchow pointed out as early as 1848 that: "History has shown more than once that the fates of the greatest empires have been decided by the health of their peoples or of their armies, and there is no longer any doubt that the history of epidemic diseases must form an inseparable part of the cultural history of mankind. Epidemics correspond to large signs of warning which tell the true statesman that a disturbance has occurred in the development of his people which even a policy of unconcern can no longer overlook."[60] It is impossible to consider here all the implications of this statement. What we can retain is the relation it suggests between epidemic diseases and the future of a state. The political history of many precolonial states can be read to good purpose in the light of this new insight, as epidemics often go hand in hand with the temporary or final subversion of the established order and the rise of new political leaders. Thus, in the Kongo kingdom, for example, in the beginning of the 18th century, several smallpox epidemics, coupled with other disasters (famines, wars) caused a general dissident movement led by a young woman. The prophetess, described in all contemporary texts as a "fetishist" and a "witch", performed miracles, healed the sick, and at the same time claimed that she would restore the power of the state, the fertility of the land and women, and the health of the people.[61] In another situation, in Central Africa again, over the last two-thirds of the XIX century, we can see chiefs and kings whose legitimacy dated from a fairly early era losing their power to new men. Several authors have interpreted this general movement, which must be associated with the upsurge in trade and the disintegration of the epidemiological landscapes discussed above, as a sort of secularization of power, as the traditional chieftains, endowed with magic and religious attributes, were unable to withstand new men whose strength lay in their material wealth, control over many dependents, and the possession of unprecedented destructive means.[62] Yet nothing is more uncertain. To take just one example, one of these new men, Mushidi, founder of the state of Garenganze in what is now Zaire, began his political move by personally inoculating the inhabitants of the region, until then defenceless, against smallpox.[63] Based on this exploit, his legitimacy went unchallenged until the very end of the XIX century, when new epidemics broke out that he was unable to control and which fatally undermined his authority. Many similar examples can be found in all the Bantu societies of southern and Central Africa. The question remains why the epidemics caused political authority to be challenged in these cases and not in the states of West Africa and central Sudan. The answer may lie in how political power was perceived, and, in particular, in the importance given to the conceptions of disease and preoccupations about health. In an ideology of sacred royalty, the most common ideology among Bantu societies, the person who holds political power is, among other things, the one who regulates nature, ensures the basic physical and biological balances, and who must account for all disturbances. As early as the 17th century, a text noted that: "When things do not go according to their wishes, if it rains too much or too little, or if other misfortunes occur, the blame is invariably placed on the king."[64] This ideology has undoubtedly existed elsewhere, for in speaking of the inhabitants of Sudan, for example, an Arab writer observed: "Their religion is the adoration of their kings and they believe that it is the kings who give them life and death, illness and health."[65] But Islam, which came to some places earlier than other, came to the rescue of political power, so to speak, by giving supreme and, during the most drastic and serious pathological crises, exclusive reign to a religious type of aetiology. Analogous aetiologies also prevailed in some West African states that were still animistic. Thus, in Dahomey, smallpox, which wreaked havoc, fitted perfectly into cosmological and religious conceptions: it was the most effective instrument of vengeance and regulation of the god Sagbata, eldest son of the primeval divine couple Mawu-Lisa, who had control over what happened on earth. Any attempt to heal or prevent smallpox would bring an immediate response from the god in the form of thunderbolts.[66]

Just as epidemic crises were a test for political leaders, periods of change, uncertainty or political tension were not without an impact on diseases and health systems. From this perspective, no period in black Africa is as illuminating as the "colonial era". Though there are no detailed studies, it is already known that the half-century during which colonial rule was being established (1880—1930) caused an unusual deterioration in general living conditions that can be clearly seen in the frequency of epidemics and the high rate of mortality. Many oral traditions gathered in very diverse regions preserve an image of this period as "the time of death". The local systems of interpretation of disease and the bio-pathological or symbolic effectiveness of therapeutic practices were severely tested, while the new medical and political authorities tried to gain as great an advantage as possible from these repeated disasters. The diseases of this period were thus the occasion of many clashes, as is shown, for example, by the 1914 plague epidemic in Dakar.[68] This epidemic, like many others that would ravage Africa after 1880, was part of the great plague pandemic which came out of Eastern Asia in about 1890. It struck Dakar in 1914 at a very unusual juncture characterized not only by increasingly heavy colonization, but also by the successful opposition to it. The epidemic was officially declared on May 13, just a few days after an African had, for the first time ever and after a bitter fight, defeated his French opponents in legislative elections. The epidemic, whose immediate effects were relatively mild, caused some 1,400 deaths in a city of about 30,000 inhabitants. It caused large demonstrations, however, until early 1915. Africans saw it in the light of two complementary and competing aetiologies: one, focusing on the rapid, fatal and abrupt development of the disease, was a religious aetiology; the other, concerned about the glaring racial inequality in the numbers of the victims (99.8% of those who died from the plague were black) took on a political character, the plague being seen as the vengeance of those defeated in the elections. There were varied reactions to an ailment caused both by God and by man: concealing of the dead; refusal to subject the bodies of the living to the diabolical manipulations of European doctors; opposition, whether passive or armed, to the classic measures of displacement and isolation. The colonials, for their part, took advantage of the displacement of populations, in theory a temporary measure carried out with the help of the army, to expropriate vast amounts of land at little cost. Above all, the idea of residential segregation, until then defended only by specialists in "colonial medicine", gained approval at all levels of European society and, thanks to the expropriations, took root in the city. Thus, the health policy of the colonial powers, often studied from a smugly triumphalist and hagiographical[69] perspective, seems to obey the logic of a system of general domination rather than that of the scattered and selfless initiatives of doctors concerned with bettering the lot of mankind.

All in all, the few directions indicated here sketch the outlines of an astonishingly rich and complex field in which disease, as the main subject of study, casts a completely new light on every nook and cranny of the social edifice. In short, faced with this new field to be conquered, it is not material that is wanting for our labours, but quite the opposite.

NOTES

1. For example, J. Christie, *Cholera Epidemics in East Africa*, London, 1876; G. Martin, *L'existence au Cameroun: études sociales, études médicales, études d'hygiène et de prophylaxie*, Paris, 1921.
2. S.M. Cissoko, "Famines et épidémies a Tombouctou et dans la Boucle du Niger du XVIe au XVIIIe siècle", *Bulletin de l'Institut fondamental d'Afrique noire* (Dakar), B. ser., XXX, pp. 806-821; J. Ford, *The Role of Trypanosomiasis in African Ecology: a Study of the Tsetse Fly Problem*, Oxford, Clarendon Press, 1971; C. Wondji, "La fièvre jaune à Grand-Bassam (1899-1903)", *Revue française d'histoire d'outre-mer*, LIX, No. 215, 1975, pp. 204-239; G.W. Hartwig and K.D. Patterson, eds., *Diseases in African History: an Introductory Survey and Case Studies*, Durham, Duke University Press, 1978.
3. L.G. Gann and Peter Duignan, *Burden of Empire: an Appraisal of Western Colonialism in Africa South of the Sahara*, London, Pall Mall Press, 1968.
4. Ibid., p. 283.
5. "They could not ... cure their patients of malaria, sleeping sickness, bilharziosis, ankylostomiasis, or other such infectious diseases. They had no remedy for onchocerciasis, conjunctivitis, tuberculosis, leprosy, rheumatism, epilepsy, diabetes or heart attacks, or for serious diseases such as typhoid, pneumonia or meningitis.... Despite all the stories, which we owe to the pens of journalists or sensationalistic writers, about mysterious and wonderful treatments, the pharmacopeia of Bantu doctors has so far given little of scientific value." (ibid., p. 283)

6. See in particular Dr. F. Sorel, *Essai de démographie des colonies françaises*, Laval, 1937.
7. Robert R. Kuczynski, *The Cameroons and Togoland: a Demographic Study*, London, 1939; *Demographic Survey of the British Colonial Empire*, Vol. I, *West Africa*, London, 1948, and Vol. II, *South Africa, High Commission Territories, East Africa*, London, 1949.
8. R.R. Kuczynski, op. cit. (1949), pp. 120-125, 144, 190-193, 235-283.
9. R.R. Kuczynski, op. cit. (1948), pp. 232-233, 239-274, 363-381, 472-521.
10. A. Romaniuk, *La fécondité des populations congolaises*, Paris, Mouton, 1967. Also see J. van Riel and R. Allard, *Contribution à l'étude de la dénatalité dans l'ethnie mongo*, Brussels, Institut royal colonial belge, 1953, and the dense and disorderly book by A. Retel-Laurentin, *Infécondité en Afrique noire: maladies et conséquences sociales*, Paris, Masson, 1974.
11. Eric de Dampierre, *Un ancien royaume Bandia au Haut-Oubangui*, Paris, Plon, 1967, pp. 111-150.
12. Giller Sautter, *De l'Atlantique au fleuve Congo: une géographie du sous-peuplement*, Paris, Mouton, 1966, 2 vol.
13. These works owe a great deal to Pierre Gourou; see in particular among his books: *La densité de la population au Rwanda Urundi, esquisse d'une etude geographique*, Brussels, Institut royal colonial belge, 1953, and *La densité de la population rurale au Congo belge*, Brussels, Acadmie royale des sciences coloniales, 1954.
14. G. Sautter, op. cit., vol. II, p. 866.
15. J.N. Biraben and J. Le Goff, "La peste dans le Haut Moyen-Age", *Annales E.S.C.*, XXIV, 6, 1969, p. 1485. Jan Vansina underscores these problems amongst the Kuba of Zaire in *The Children of Woot: a History of the Kuba Peoples*, Madison, University of Wisconsin Press, 1978, p. 85.
16. J. Ford has also shown that the Europeans, at the beginnings of colonization, did not understand at all the terrible epizootic of 1889-1896, which decimated up to 80% of the herds. According to Ford, that is why contemporary colonial texts make no mention of the catastrophe (cf. J. Ford, op. cit., p. 141).
17. S.M. Cissoko, op. cit., pp. 814-820; M. Tymowski, *Le développement et la régression chez les peuples de la Boucle du Niger à l'époque pré-coloniale*, Warsaw, Universitytet Warszawski, Institut Historyczny, 1974.
18. These were in fact epidemics of other, unidentified, diseases. Only the epidemic of 1741-43 could have been the plague, since it had by that time reached the bend of the Niger from Morocco, where it was then raging (cf. S.M. Cissoko, op. cit. p. 818).
19. Tymowski, "Famines et epidemies a Oualatta et a Tichit au XIXe siecle", *Africana Bulletin* (Warsaw), No. 27, 1978, pp. 35-53.
20. Unless otherwise indicated, the information is from the National Archives, (Overseas Section), Senegal series, XI, 30.
21. C. Pulvenis de Séligny, "La fièvre jaune en Afrique occidentale il y a cent ans", *Afrique médicale* (Dakar), XV, 1976, No. 143, pp. 581-588, and No. 144, pp. 669-672.

22. See in particular Dr. F. Cazanove, "Histoire épidémique de la fièvre jaune", *Outre-mer*, 2nd quarter, 1930, pp. 160-180.

23. Dr. Auvray and Dr. Boury, "Rapport sur l'épidémie de fièvre jaune qui a régné au Soudan français en 1897", *Annales d'hygiène et de médicine coloniales*, I, 1898, pp. 433-464.

24. Dr. A. Kermogant, "Epidémie de fièvre jaune au Sénégal du 16 avril 1900 au 28 fevrier 1901", *Annales d'hygiène et de médicine coloniales*, V, 1901, pp. 413-414.

25. Cazanove, op. cit., p. 173.

26. See for example H.M. Feinberg, "New data on European mortality in West Africa: the Dutch on the Gold Coast, 1719-1760", *Journal of African History*, XV, 1974, pp. 357-371; K.G. Davies, "The living and the dead: white mortality in West Africa, 1684-1732", in S.L. Engerman and E.D. Genovese, eds., *Race and Slavery in the Western Hemisphere: Quantitative Studies*, Princeton, Princeton University Press, 1975, pp. 83-93. This also applies to the minorities of black slaves returned from America: see R. Kuczynski, op. cit. (1948), pp. 40-153, 197-207 (for Sierra Leone), and T.W. Shick, "A quantitative analysis of Liberian colonisation from 1820 to 1843 with special reference to mortality", *Journal of African History*, XII, 1971, pp. 45-59.

27. On this view, see P.D. Curtin, "The white man's grave: image and reality, 1780-1850", *Journal of British Studies*, I, 1961, pp. 94-110, and *The Image of Africa: British Ideas and Action, 1780-1850*, Madison, University of Wisconsin Press, 1964.

28. His major publications in the medical field are *The Medical Topography of the West Coast of Africa*, London, 1859; *The Diseases of Tropical Climates and their Treatment*, London, 1874. See C. Fyfe, *Africanus Horton, 1835-1883: West African Scientist and Patriot*, London, Oxford University Press, 1972.

29. One of the best examples is J. Ringenbuch and Dr. Guyomarc'h, "Notes de géographie médicale de la section française de la mission de délimitation Afrique Equatoriale Française --Cameroun (1912-1913)", *Bulletin de la Société de pathologie exotique*, VIII, 1915, pp. 129-130, 199-208, 301-313, 515-546.

30. For Dakar, for example: Dr. C. Jopot, *Dakar, essai de géographie médicale et d'ethnographie*, Mondidier, 1907, and Dr. G. Ribot and R. Lafon, *Dakar, ses origines, son avenir*, Paris, 1908.

31. G. Martin, op. cit., p. 3.

32. M.D. Grmek, "Géographie médicale et histoire des civilisations", *Annales E.S.C.*, XVIII, 1963, pp. 1071-1097.

33. This notion, though less evocative than the Anglo-American *disease environment*, seems preferable to the notion of *pathocenose* proposed by M.D. Grmek and which refers to the same thing. See G. Remy, ed., *Introductions épidémiologiques à une étude géographique des maladies en Afrique tropicale*, Marseille, EHESS, Centre pluridisciplinaire de la Vieille Charité, 1979 (multigr.); M.D. Grmek, "Préliminaires d'une étude historique des maladies", *Annales E.S.C.*, XXIV, 6, 1969, pp. 1473-1483.

34. M. Gluckman, "The individual in a social framework: the rise of king Shaka of Zululand", *Journal of African Studies*, I, 1974, pp. 113-144; J.D. Omer-Cooper, *The Zulu Aftermath: a Nineteenth Century Revolution in Bantu Africa*, London, Longman, 1966; J. Guy, "Ecological factors in the rise of Shaka and

the Zulu kingdom" in S. Marks and A. Atmore, eds., *Economy and Society in Pre-Industrial South Africa*, London, Longman, 1980, pp. 102-119.

35. This is only conjecture, based especially on accounts of travels that are difficult to interpret because the nosographical pictures they paint may be linked to the situation arising from repeated contact with Europeans. See G. Sautter, op. cit., vol. II, pp. 996-999; E. M'Bokolo, *Noirs et Blancs en Afrique équatoriale. Les sociétés côtières et la pénétration française (vers 1820-1874)*, Paris, Mouton, 1981, p. 17; J. Vansina, "The peoples of the forest", in D. Birmingham and P. Martin, eds., *History of Central Africa*, Vol. I, London, Longman (at press).

36. See in particular R. Oliver and B.M. Fagan, *Africa in the Iron Age (c. 500 B.C. to A.D. 1400)*, Cambridge University Press, 1975, pp. 29-32, 70-80, 106-118, 203.

37. J.D. Omer-Cooper, op. cit., pp. 99-114.

38. C. Chamberlin, "The migration of the Fang into Central Gabon during the nineteenth century", *International Journal of African Historical Studies*, XI, 1978, pp. 429-456; E. M'Bokolo, op. cit., pp. 136-138, 194; K.D. Patterson, "The vanishing Mpngwe: European contact and demographic change in the Gabon river", *Journal of African History*, XVI, 1975, pp. 217-238.

39. From indications in J.C. Miller, "The Atlantic zone from 1400 to 1870: the paradoxes of impoverishment", in D. Birmingham and P. Martin, eds., op. cit. Also see R. Hoeppli, "Parasitic diseases in Africa and the western hemisphere: early documentation and transmission by the slave trade", *Acta Tropica* (Basel), supplement 10, 1969.

40. Several recent studies touch on this question. See in particular: G.W. Hartwig, *The Art of Survival in East Africa: the Kerebe and Long-Distance Trade, 1800-1895*, New York, Africana Publishing Company, 1976 (and the very good summary by S. Feierman in the *International Journal of African Historical Studies*, XII, 1979, pp. 653-672); H. Kjekshus, *Ecology of Control and Economic Development in East African History: the Case of Tanganyika 1850-1950*, London, Heinemann, 1977; John Iliffe, *A Modern History of Tanganyika*, Cambridge University Press, 1978; B.A. Ogot, ed., *Ecology and History in East Africa*, Nairobi, Kenya Literature Bureau, 1979.

41. R. Gray and D. Birmingham, eds., *Precolonial African Trade. Essays on Trade in Central and Eastern Africa before 1900*, Oxford University Press, 1970.

42. J. Christie, op. cit.

43. S.M. Cissoko, op. cit., and J.R. Dias, "Famine and disease in the history of Angola, c. 1830-1930", *Journal of African History*, XXII, 1981, pp. 349-378.

44. H. Kjekshus, op. cit., pp. 9-25, and "The population trends of East African history: a critical review", in *African Historical Demography*, Edinburg, Centre of African Studies, 1977, pp. 352-362; R.M.A. Van Zwanenberg and A. King, *An Economic History of Kenya and Uganda 1800-1970*, London, Macmillan, 1975, pp. 3-7, 110-122, 145-159; J. Iliffe, op. cit., pp. 67-77.

45. G.H. Hartwig, op. cit.

46. G.W. Hartwig, "Long-distance trade and the evolution of sorcery among the Kerebe", *International Journal of African Historical Studies*, IV, 1971, pp. 505-524.

47. J. Iliffe, op. cit.

48. J.M. Janzen, "Ideologies and institutions in the precolonial history of equatorial African therapeutic systems", *Social Science and Medicine*, XIII, part B, No. 4, 1979, p. 318.

49. J.M. Jamzen (with W. Arkinstall), *The Quest for Therapy in Lower Zaire*, Berkeley, University of California Press, 1978, p. 8, 67, 74.

50. Ibid., p. 11, 37-65; S. Feierman, "Change in African therapeutic systems", *Social Science and Medicine*, XIII, part B, No. 4, 1979, pp. 277-284; G. Prins, "Disease at the crossroads: towards a history of therapeutics in Bulozi since 1876", *Social Science and Medicine*, XIII, part B, No. 4, 1979, pp. 285-315.

51. This is the *therapy managing group*, a concept which Janzen, Feierman and Prins (op. cit.) make great use of in their works.

52. J. Vansina, op. cit., pp. 197-210.

53. E.W. Herbert, "Smallpox inoculation in Africa", *Journal of African History*, XVI, 1975, pp. 539-559.

54. F. Quinn, "How traditional Dahomean society interpreted smallpox", *Abbia* (Yaounde), No. 20, 1968, pp. 151-166.

55. D. Maier, "Nineteenth-century Asante medical practices", *Comparative Studies in Society and History*, XXI, 1979, pp. 63-81.

56. Ivor Wilks, *Asante in the Nineteenth Century. The Structure and Evolution of a Political Order*, Cambridge University Press, 1975.

57. J. Janzen, op. cit.; P. Martin, *The External Trade of the Loango Coast, 1576-1870*, Oxford, Clarendon Press, 1972.

58. J. Janzen, op. cit., p. 319.

59. A.J.H. Latham, "Witchcraft accusations and economic tension in precolonial Old Calabar", *Journal of African History*, XIII, 1972, pp. 319-360.

60. Quoted by René Dubos, *Man Adapting*, New Haven, 1965. I would like to thank Claudine Herzlich for giving me this reference.

61. L. Jadin, "Le Congo et la secte des Antoniens. Restauration du royaume sous Pedro IV et la Saint Antoine congolaise, 1604-1718", *Bulletin de l'Institut historique belge de Rome*, XXXIII, 1961, pp. 411-614.

62. P. Curtin, S. Feierman, L. Thompson and J. Vansina, *African History*, London, Longman, 1978, pp. 391-417.

63. E. M'Bokolo, *Msiri*, Dakar, Nouvelles éditions africaines, Paris, ABC, 1976.

64. O. Dapper, *Description de l'Afrique* (Amsterdam, 1686), quoted by W.G.L. Randles, *L'ancien royaume du Congo des origines à la fin du XIXe siècle*, Paris, Mouton, 1968, p. 33.

65. W.G.L. Randles, ibid., p. 33, n. 2.

66. F. Quinn, op. cit., pp. 155-156; Melville J. Herskovits, *Dahomey, an Ancient West African Kingdom*, New York, J.-J. Augustin, 1938, Vol. 2, pp. 135-137.

67. P. Curtin, et al., op. cit., pp. 552-555.

68. Studied in detail in E. M'Bokolo, "Peste et société urbaine à Dakar: l'épidémie en 1914", *Cahiers d'études africaines* (to be published soon).

69. See for example L.H. Gann and P. Duignan, op. cit.; J.J. McKelvey, *Man against Tsetse: Struggle for Africa*, Ithaca, Cornell University Press, 1973, and the abundant general literature on the great colonial and tropicalist physicians.

FROM THE RIGHT TO ILLNESS TO THE DUTY TO BE HEALTHY: THE INDUSTRIAL SOCIETY

Part II

FROM THE RIGHT TO
ILLNESS TO THE DUTY
TO BE HEALTHY:
THE INDUSTRIAL SOCIETY

Chapter 5

MODERN MEDICINE AND THE QUEST FOR MEANING. ILLNESS AS A SOCIAL SIGNIFIER

C. Herzlich

All societies strive to find a connection between the biological order and the social order. In all societies, illness can be connected to causes of a social nature. How is this connection made in our society? What do we mean when we speak, and we do so more and more often, about the "social dimension" of illness? Since the 1950s in the United States, and since the late 1960s in France, sociology has begun to answer these questions.

These questions are, for sociology, both paradoxical and highly important. Paradoxical because illness, health and death are highly "natural", "physical", and "objective" subjects, so that they seem at first to fall outside the realm of social reality: it is impossible to ignore the "physical" evidence of illness, old age, and death, and that evidence seems to sum up their entire existence. But they are also highly important because it becomes all the more essential to show how they are indissolubly linked to social reality in many ways.

Illness is first of all a social fact. There are different kinds of illnesses, and they are differently distributed depending on the period, the society, and social conditions. We have many examples of this: the "epidemics", "fevers", and "phthisis" of the past have been replaced in the West today by cardiovascular disease and cancer. Some infectious diseases which are benign in our countries and are becoming rare still take a heavy toll in third world countries. In France even today, the life expectancy of teachers, executives, and members of the liberal professions is several years longer than for manual labourers, etc.

However, it was not sociologists but, long before them, a trend in medicine, social hygiene, which first regarded illness as a social fact and tried throughout the 18th and 19th centuries with a certain measure of success to establish its causes in social terms. "Medical topographies" and studies on social hygiene were forerunners to the work of today's epidemiologists. They clearly linked the health of a population to its living conditions, which were themselves determined by its social position. Social hygiene or "social medicine" was developed in all the major European countries. In France, Villermé studied everything from the health problems of textile workers to the relationship between mortality and poverty in different parts of Paris or the duration of an illness depending on social factors. In Germany, Virchow pointed out the economic, social and political causes, the influence of the Church in particular, of the 1847 typhus epidemic in Silesia. The work of social hygienists also led to political action. It was because of Virchow's action that Germany established its system of social and medical insurance at the end of the 19th century. Similarly in England, Chadwick played an important role in the establishment of the British institutions of social medicine.

At the end of the 19th century, however, the discoveries of Pasteur and with them the theory of "specific aetiology" (that each disease is caused by a specific germ) usurped the territory occupied by social hygiene. It did not disappear, but instead acquired the means to become even more effective, though it was relegated to second place in science. The idea of specific aetiology and the discovery of the germs causing many illnesses led to the development of various types of effective prophylactic measures. The sterilization of milk beginning in the 1890s allowed infantile diarrhoea, which at the time was causing the deaths of large numbers of small infants, to be brought under control; the introduction of asepsis and then antisepsis into hospital services significantly reduced post-surgical mortality; typhoid was brought under control thanks to public works for the supply of unpolluted drinking water, and so on.

Social hygiene was thus more active than ever. The battles against the "plagues of society", tuberculosis, alcoholism, syphilis, mobilized large sectors of society through various leagues, associations and campaigns. In many cases, however, these battles became an excuse for government intervention and social control: the "germ bearer" was supposedly being neutralized when in fact the working class was being stigmatized. In 1902, the public health law, which advocates of social hygiene had been demanding for several decades, was a decisive stage in what would later be called the "medicalization of society".

However, to medical thinking itself, social variables were henceforth considered secondary causes of illness. They were simply the circumstances which made a germ or a disease more or less widespread in a given place at a given time. The inscribing of the germ's effect on the individual body became the essential thing; the distribution of the condition in geographico-social space seemed secondary. In 1893, after the discovery of the Koch bacillus, Emile Behring wrote that the struggle against infectious diseases could now be pursued unswervingly without being sidetracked by social considerations.[1] Despite its success, or perhaps because of it, because a certain number of problems could be controlled by routine technical means, the social hygiene trend became less important in medicine. Public health, social hygiene, and social medicine became minor specialities; at the same time, public health doctors became a sub-group commanding little esteem within the medical profession.

I THE MEDICAL CONSTRUCTION OF ILLNESS

Around 1950, in the United States, the nascent sociology of medicine declared itself the offspring of the social hygiene and social medicine of the 19th century. In fact that was only partially true, and the claim that Villermé, Virchow and Chadwick were its founding fathers had more to do with the tendency of all newly emerging professional groups to gain legitimacy by asserting a direct link with great ancestors. As a matter of fact, sociologists have done little work on the problem of the social causes of illness and, despite a few brilliant exceptions,[2] have made only a small contribution to the development of social epidemiology. It is also striking that those who have worked on it did not, until recently,[3] challenge the framework of the clinical entities recognized by medical thought, and have not developed a purely sociological conception of aetiology. On the contrary, they have studied *illness as social behaviour*. The social status and the role of the sick person in our society, the variables which determine his conduct and the norms which shape it, and his relations with the medical institution, have been the subject-matter par excellence of the hundreds of studies which, over the past 30 years, have called themselves "medical sociology".[4]

It is possible, if we accept the simplification involved in all classifications of this type, to distinguish two trends which differ in the status they grant to knowledge and medical conceptions and to their legitimacy and exclusive authority for defining illness. As can be seen from Marc Augé's article, anthropology too has encountered these problems, there too several approaches can be distinguished which view in different ways the relation between the traditional conceptions of disease within a given group and the conceptions developed by Western medicine. While we are well aware of how pertinent this problem is to societies other than our own, it may seem irrelevant for us, since on the whole we hold medicine to be the "truth". The problem exists nevertheless. There is no real reason, and in any event it is not a foregone conclusion, why in our society any more than in another everyone should identify disease entirely and exclusively with the medical view of it. If this were the case, doctors would be less inclined to complain about their patients and patients about their doctors.

In the 1950s, however, the first sociologists to study illness adopted and fully accepted the medical conceptions of pathological phenomena: disease was a biochemical process affecting the individual body. Health and illness were in themselves organic realities independent of place and time and of the characteristics of the individuals and groups concerned. From this objectivity of disorders came the conception of medical knowledge as a reading of the organic state, a decoding which scientific progress was making daily more exact and accurate. We could say that the basis of this underlying conception of many studies is the notion of the *legitimacy of medicine in decoding an organic state*. According to this notion, medical concepts enable that state to be read with greater or lesser subtlety and precision but aim only at reflecting its objective reality.

Yet that reality has *social dimensions*: the circumstances, the organizational and interactional context of illness. The sociologist was to take on the task of defining what happened before, after, and around a medically defined reality. The "social dimension" of illness thus became assimilated to a series of contextual variables which had to be explored. But disease was also a social thing in its consequences: for Talcott Parsons,[5] who was the first to conceive of illness as social behaviour, illness was above all deviance because it forced the individual to become inactive. According to this viewpoint, linked to the economic point of view, man is defined as a producer, and the sick person is considered deviant because he is unproductive. All of the mechanisms attached to the patient-doctor "roles" aim at reducing that deviance and reintegrating the patient into the rounds and exchanges of social conformity which by and large amount to seeking and accepting treatment.

It is therefore not surprising that, for those sociologists who held that notion, "illness behaviour",[6] which is tantamount to *seeking medical care*, was a preferential field of study. Research consisted firstly of determining the social variables which decided whether or not treatment was sought. The few studies of "lay" conceptions of illness[7] were also meant primarily to determine the differences between those conceptions and medical knowledge, considered potential sources of resistance to seeking treatment. Seeking help was seen as expressing both rationality about health, since it led to recovery, and social rationality, it reintegrated the individual into society.

For the sociologist, the extension of his field of study to "illness behaviour" has on the whole been a success. The social context seems as important for predicting an individual's behaviour as the character or seriousness of his ailment. Moreover, this analysis can be said to correspond to many aspects of social functioning as we know it. It is true that the sick person is often *considered a deviant*. It is also true that the sick person's "desire to recover", and thus to return to his place in production, as perceived by health care practitioners, is often one of the criteria in the therapeutic management of the individual and the legitimation of his condition. But we can also see that this view, centred on a conception of man as a producer, is not itself "natural" and must be resituated within a certain state of social relations.

The many criticisms of medicine in the last decades and the revelation that there are limits to its efficacy[8] also lead us to doubt the absolute rationality of seeking treatment as postulated in this model: we now doubt whether seeking care to as great an extent and as early as possible and in every case is the best answer, and feel that avoiding it is not always deviant. Finally, on another level, we find that this model conceals the difference between the pathogenic risks run by the different social classes. One might ask whether the social classes most affected by illness, as evidenced by much epidemiological data, should by that very fact be considered more "deviant". *In fact*, this question is often answered in the affirmative: the individual's biological status is actually linked to his social status, and the same is true for social classes and social groups. *In theory*, however, the question remains.

In opposition to this line of study, a second trend has developed which could be called an approach to *medicine as producing social categories of health and illness*. For the partisans of this conception,[9] the organic reality of illness and its social reality, that is to say, the organic state in itself and the organic state defined as illness by medicine and the physician, must not be confused. They are not mere copies or continuities of each other. Various epidemiological studies have shown that many "symptoms" exist permanently in a "normal" population without causing "illness". Medical knowledge is more than a reading, then. It is a process of constructing illness as a social situation marked by deviance. A doctor does not simply put into words a state of illness that is obvious in itself, he creates it by applying the notion of a norm that has been vitiated. He names the biological deviance and in doing so creates the social deviance.[10] Social iatrogenics and medicine, says Eliot Freidson, are consubstantial.

Since medical conceptions of pathological states are not identical to a "reality", "lay" conceptions take on a certain positivity and a role in the social construction of illness.[11] Given the weight of medicine, however, the process of marking or labelling a symptom as "illness" by medicine and physicians becomes the sociologist's main subject-matter of study. He wants to understand why some states are labelled as illness and others are not, and the consequences of that fact. He must then study how illness comes to exist as a social reality, and how it is structured in the relations among individuals and groups and particularly, in treatment, the medical management of illness. This double off-centring of the analysis (the "reality" of pathological phenomena as the "truth" of medical knowledge, and the efficacy of practice, are also included here) thus aims at showing how medicine arises from social facts and in turn produces social facts.

This type of analysis has been applied successfully to the aspects of organic phenomena that are apparently most difficult to deal with sociologically, such as pain, for example. Anselm Strauss and S.Y. Fagerhaugh[12] have analyzed, from observation of different types of hospital services, the management of pain in a medical environment. It is carried out through complex processes in which the demands, organization, routines and rhythms of hospitals, the ideology of hospital and medical staff, and the negotiations between the patient, his family, and health practitioners are all expressed. The "categories" and "trajectories" of pain thus determined, and which in fact make up the reality of the patient's experiences, are not nearly so much "objective" organic characteristics of pain as a retranscribing of it as a social reality through a host of interpretations and interactions.

Until recently, such studies have, however, remained only too rare, and this trend deserves a certain amount of criticism for not having entirely transcended the programmatic stage. Researchers have long tended to avoid the "heaviest" cases of clearly organic, serious illness and have kept to the areas of mental illness[13] or the medicalization of society, easier to deal with from their point of view, but also less fruitful. There are also limits to the extent to which researchers can study medicine without referring to the positivity of its knowledge or the effectiveness of its practices as sheer symbolic response or pure ideology. Such studies can in fact shed light on certain social functions of medicine, but they cannot elucidate its actual functioning.

The study of medicine as creating social categories of health and illness should therefore try to examine the "heavy" cases of even the most somatic illnesses. Nor should it minimize the reality and efficacy of medical practice. An attempt might be made to formulate a few of the principles which could guide this type of approach.

1   It is important not to study medical knowledge from a positivistic outlook as a clearly defined, closed, and totally "objective" body of knowledge. Various studies[14] show that it is by no means devoid of what R.C. Fox has called "scientific magic". That fact could form a bridge with the anthropological study of so-called primitive medicine. Moreover, it should be considered that medical knowledge, as actually used by a given practitioner, always takes us back to the physician's place in the entire medical institution and the role of that institution within society as a whole. A study by I. Baszanger,[15] for example, shows clearly that young general practitioners are not passive receivers and users of an intangible body of medical knowledge acquired at university once and for all. During their first years of practice they actively and selectively construct systems of categories and notions through which they apprehend the illnesses and patients they are dealing with, and organize their diagnoses and therapies. These systems, which in fact represent the "operative" knowledge of general medicine, are decided by the professional ideologies of young physicians, by how they see the position of general medicine as compared to specialized and/or hospital medicine, and by their conceptions of the general practitioner's role in society.

2   In medical knowledge and practice, biological, social and ethical categories overlap in complex ways. This complex meshing is becoming increasingly intricate with the development of modern, plurilinear theories of illness, which bring into play a series of interacting factors among which psychism, the environment, and social behaviour each have their place. An extreme, sometimes

caricatural example of this meshing can be found in cases where the creation of a new nosological category, the definition of a syndrome or "illness" clearly seems to be a vehicle of social values. Thus, in France, in 1902, four years after the enactment of the 1898 law granting compensation to workers injured at work, Dr. Brissaud, a well known psychiatrist, described a new "disease", "injury syndrome",[16] or the peculiar inability of injured workers on workman's compensation to recover from their injuries. According to Dr. Brissaud, they were not malingering: the worker really was sick, but was sick because of compensation. To a degree proportionate to the seriousness of his organic state, a patient recovered or did not recover depending on whether or not he was insured. Similarly, in 1928, when the draft bill on social insurance was under debate, the case of "insurance neurosis" was raised, with illustrative statistics.

In this case, the interpretation given to an organic state is imbued with the meaning attached to the social context in which it arose. The fact that workers were paid "insurance" in the event of an accident at work, something which much of the middle class, including doctors, disapproved of, is seen as a cause of illness. A blow to dominant social values led to the creation of the entity called "injury syndrome".[16] Conversely, the true nature of an organic state can long go unrecognized due to resistance where, once again, social values are at stake. Such was the case of what is now called "child-beating". In 1879, Dr. Tardieu described "subdural haematoma of the infant", usually very serious (it was discovered during autopsies on the infants) and often accompanied by "unexplained multiple fractures". For nearly a century studies on cases of this kind were published and the syndrome was considered to be idiopathic. It was only in 1966, with the work of Dr. Neyman, that the notion of "child-beating" was accepted in France. Despite many troubling facts, doctors for decades failed to recognize that the child's condition was the result of trauma: parental mistreatment could not be conceived of by an ideology which held that any parent must needs be a good parent.

3   These examples represent extreme cases, but they aptly demonstrate how medicine can inscribe social values onto bodies, so to speak. Through diagnosis, classification and treatment of illness, medicine creates or legitimates social statuses. Here again, a few rules of analysis may be useful to specify how it does this:

   —Labelling a state as "illness" is not a socially neutral process, and in the medical management of illness there is a fine line between legitimacy and stigma. Medicine long failed to recognize the psychological and social consequences of labelling illness and felt that while diagnosis and treatment could sometimes be of no use, they could never be harmful. Hence the medical rule that it is better to mistakenly diagnose a healthy man as sick than a sick man as healthy.[17] We now know that the suspicion that he may be sick has immediate consequences for a person's identity and labelling an illness, even if erroneously, can be enough to start an individual off on a career as a sick person. Finally, we know that although illness has been granted legitimacy, everyone has the right to be ill, the sick person cannot always avoid being stigmatized.

—The special value attached to "treatment" as such in our society must also be recognized, and it can be argued that treatment, as a prescribed, obligatory response to illness, a sick person *must* seek treatment, is ascribed greater legitimacy than illness. But it can also be seen that while the existence of a recognized model of care, a routine pattern of therapeutic action, legitimates the pathological condition it is meant to treat, the absence of such a model tends to render the pathological condition illegitimate. The "functionally ill", the incurables for whom no known therapy exists, tend to be not only abandoned medically, but even rejected both psychologically and socially.

—Though they appear most often to be the subjects, even the victims, of the professional's work, the sick are actually parties to these social relations and play an active role in them. This is especially true for the cases, more and more common today, of the chronically ill whose long "careers" as patients lead to a great deal of experience and highly developed knowledge about their ailments. Some diabetics, for example, know more about diabetes than a general practitioner. Patients such as these actively negotiate the management of their condition with their doctors, and take part in the "social construction of illness". In England and the United States, a great deal of research has been done on these subjects in the past few years. *There is a recognition of the active role of the patient and the importance of lay conceptions.* But perhaps not all of the implications of this phenomenon have been recognized. To take lay thinking about illness fully into account is not a matter of simply adding an extra dimension to the analysis, but implies, we believe, *another conception of the connections between illness and social reality.* It is this idea that we shall now examine.

II ILLNESS AS A SIGNIFIER

In assuming the task of studying the mechanisms and consequences of the medical construction of illness, sociology has recognized that in our society illness is the "business" of medicine alone and that the ties it once had with, for example, religion, the family, and the kinship system, ties which still exist in other societies, have loosened considerably.

In doing so, however, sociology has left out another problem: today illness is in fact in the hands of medicine, but it continues to overflow into many other areas. Busy explaining how a biological process affecting a person's body is defined and treated by the physician, concentrating on how this happens and the effects it has, sociologists have forgotten the other face of illness. For all of us, illness is not just the set of symptoms which prompts us to consult a doctor; it is still the unfortunate event that threatens or irremediably changes our individual lives, or a collective disaster with incalculable consequences.[18] Seen thus, illness always demands an interpretation that goes beyond the individual body and specific aetiology. It always entails questions about its *causes* (which in our minds cannot be reduced to a germ or genetic factors), and even more so about its *meaning*:[19] "why me?", "why him?", "why here?", "why now?" The medical information we share in, the diagnoses offered by the practitioner and accepted by us are usually not enough to answer those questions. Furthermore, it would be wrong to think that this need to interpret illness, to assign it causes conceived of in non-organic terms, to give it a meaning, are basically a relic from the days when, scientific medicine not yet having provided the "real" answers, man created meanings to fill the breaches in his knowledge. We believe on the contrary that this need, though it now takes specific forms, is as strong as ever. Far from coming into play only where medicine fails, it includes everything connected to the body and human life in a collective discourse that has its own logic independent of medical models. What elements of medical information it contains gain their meaning firstly from being placed within a different language, that of the individual-society relationship.

The collective interpretation of illness is made in terms which, in the strict sense of the wording, *challenge society or the social order*. Illness, Susan Sontag rightly said, is a "metaphor".[20] Through our conceptions of illness we are in fact talking about something else: society and our relations to it. Because it requires interpretation, illness thus becomes a basis of meaning, a signifier whose signified is the individual's relationship with the social order. These questions and their answers may remain comparatively secondary for the physician. They should be of prime importance to the sociologist. This is true first and foremost because, as in societies other than our own where people know how very important thought on illness can be in "ideo-logic",[21] illness affords us access to beliefs, interpretations, values, all the relations of meaning being formed in our society. Secondly, and this does not contradict but instead does complement our previous analyses, our approach to medicine and its impact on our culture may be revitalized by these questions: certainly medicine shapes illness, and this is undoubtedly peculiar to our society, but it must nevertheless, reciprocally, itself be apprehended in the framework of our relationship with society, based on the views of illness that make it a metaphor.

This problem has been partially dealt with in France through the study of the social representations of health and illness. The idea was to show that there is a coherent system of thought, a separate system of conceptions of health and illness independent of the categories of medical knowledge. This study shows clearly that the language used to express health and illness is not a language of the body, of organic facts, it is a language of the individual's relationship with the socialized exterior, with society. In a study of members of the middle class, management, and the liberal professions done in the 1960s,[22] we showed that activity or inactivity, social participation or exclusion, are the notions that are constantly used to define the sick and the healthy person. "I've never been sick, I've never been off work", was heard time and again from people asked to describe their experience of illness. This reference defines illness better than any allusion to a bodily state. Collective discourse is thus not a more or less exact copy of medical discourse and its notions, a list of symptoms and bodily processes. On the contrary, symptoms, dysfunctions, take on meaning and become organized into an "illness" only in so far as they introduce some change into the life and social identity of the sick person. These are also the criteria by which the degree of seriousness of an organic state can be determined and, especially, by which the very meaning of the sick person's experience is defined. Illness is experienced as "destructive" when the affected person sees no possibility of recovering his identity, which is wholly equated with social integration. It is "liberating", on the other hand, when he perceives illness as a chance to escape a social role that is stifling his individuality. In "illness as an occupation", finally, the individual retains his identity. To him illness corresponds to a specific but lasting social integration: the "sick role" is a social role.

Correlatively, from the aetiological point of view, illness in its genesis is attributed to a society that is "aggressive" and "constraining" because it imposes an unhealthy "lifestyle" on the individual. People enumerate *ad infinitum* the unhealthy elements which in large quantities cause illness: air pollution, adulterated and "chemical" food, noise, the hectic pace of life. Illness thus embodies and crystallizes social aggression, and social aggression is interpreted as present or future illness. In contrast to society, the individual is characterized in terms of health, a greater or lesser potential for resisting aggression. The individual is fundamentally healthy, and health is entirely an individual thing. The representation of health and illness can thus be schematized as two sets of opposites: the health-illness antithesis duplicates and objectifies the individual-society antithesis. Within this framework, the sick person is a sort of symbolic figure: he is the exemplary victim of the forces bearing upon us.

This representation contains themes that appear far back in history. Polluted air, for example, was cited as a cause of the plague as early as the Middle Ages. What we find above all, however, in modern form, is a classic schema in anthropology wherein exogenous illness is brought on by an exterior cause, by the real or symbolic intrusion of a harmful object, one of the key notions of the representation is that of "poisoning", meaning the slow but steady intake of harmful elements and, at a more general level, the maleficent acts of an unhealthy entity, society. The representation of the genesis of illness is more complex, however. The individual plays an essential part in it through his "resistance", his "strength" and "healthiness". The individual has some part of responsibility for an illness that is entirely society-induced. The representation serves to set out the relations, and the conflicts, between them.

The striking thing here is that a representation such as this expresses a view of a "society" that is not conceived of as a set of social interactions. It is not apprehended through the relations or conflicts of different groups but through an objectifying of it as a harmful environment, air pollution, noise, unhealthy food. Such a representation is thus subject to a certain "neutralization": the social reality involved is one not of power relations but of environmental conditions. It is made something natural by being expressed in terms of concrete environmental conditions. Poisoning represents the inscribing of these harmful physical elements on the body of a particular individual, on his resistance, his specific state of health. The representation thus brings us face to face with a society viewed as an overall entity with primarily physical manifestations, and isolated individuals somewhat removed from social relations: it sees illness first as the illness of an isolated individual. We might therefore find it remarkable that, despite the importance given to the idea of activity, occupational illnesses as a threat to groups with the same working conditions are practically absent from the representation. On the other hand, ample mention is made of "psychological" illnesses, bringing into play individual intrapsychical processes.[23] Similarly, while the longer individual lifespan and differences in life expectancies depending on social category are frequently commented on, the fact that different social classes have differential risks of illness did not figure in the collective representation of the 1960s, at least among the middle classes.[24]

We might also note the connection between these conceptions and the actual pathology of a period on one hand, and on the other, the system of collective relations which gradually institutionalizes around illness. During the 1960s, the prevailing representation was that of an individual illness, and it is true that, compared to previous eras, illness has today become *individualized*. What was once the predominating disease, the collective plague, the epidemic which never strikes the individual but always the community, has disappeared from Western countries. Classic descriptions of the plague always mention the large number of deaths and the breakdown of social order. Today, not only has the plague disappeared in fact, but it has also been erased from memory.[25] The overriding image of illness is that of an individual attack. The fact that someone is ill does not mean that others are ill: a person is ill alone. At the same time, however, illness has become *socialized* with the emergence of a collective form of management by social legislation. Work, activity, played an essential role in this development. During the 19th century, with industrial development, health came to mean the ability to work, and illness, the inability to do so. This connection, operative within the representation, does indeed correspond to a reality, but it is not a "natural" connection, it is socio-historical. In response to a pressing problem, the need to care for the ill and to restore health as a condition for production, the system of social insurance was gradually introduced and in France it reached its final form in 1945. Every wage-earner, by virtue of his employment, was insured for medical care and loss of income in the event of illness. Illness became a legitimate, socially recognized reason for inactivity.

Throughout the 20th century, the problem of health has thus been posed in collective terms, as part of the social question. Faced with industrial exploitation, workers demanded working conditions compatible with health, access to medical care, and compensation for illness or industrial accident. The most clear-sighted doctors, for their part, realized that by accepting social insurance they could make a profit from the poor, whom they had hitherto treated as charitable cases. Through insurance and social legislation, illness and medicine did indeed take on a collective dimension, but illness was then individualized in another way: it would henceforth be treated in the individual doctor-patient relationship. The patient-work connection was highly important, but it would be expressed in an individual's stopping work at the instance of another individual, and would involve those two alone. Social relations became somewhat neutralized by being medicalized. As we have seen, representations of illness bore even recently the marks of this fact.

What we have tried to show is that, deeply embedded in social reality, "lay" representations of health and illness are by no means reducible to medical conceptions of pathological facts. They are not an impoverishment or distortion of those facts. They occupy another level and answer different questions. Yet they are not isolated for all that, and can incorporate many elements from medical knowledge. As a result, medicine is also less independent than it would appear from the collective discourse. It is by taking these two levels of analysis into account that sociology could apprehend the social construction of health and illness in its entirety.

Such an analysis is, we feel, a task of crucial importance today. Studies done since the first work on social representations[26] show that the basic dimensions, the logic governing them, have in essence remained unchanged: the individual is still expressing his relation to social reality through his view of biological illness. But the very meaning of these representations within our society, *the importance of illness, health, and the body as metaphorical objects, as bases for the meaning of our relation to society, has, in our opinion, increased substantially* and its content has become specific. Today, our view of illness and the institution which manages it, medicine, is in some way at the epicentre of cultural and social conflicts. It no longer merely reflects the image of a harmful society inflicting even physical damage on the individual. It crystallizes some of our questions and our most acute anxieties about two of the salient characteristics of social evolution: the growing importance of science and technology on one hand, and the widespread movement towards professionalization on the other.

The antitheses in the representation remain the same, but they have developed to include new aspects. The individual, his body, his health, and his harmony with nature, are still fundamental assets threatened by an aggressive society. However, and this is a new element connected to the development of new medical technology and the movements towards medicalization in our society, *medicine has itself become one of the major expressions of "social reality", its constraints and dangers*. In the 1960s, the individual was integrated into society or felt himself excluded by reason of his health or illness. Today his relation to illness has become, more exclusively than in the past, a relationship with medicine, with "professional" health care management and with a body of knowledge and practices bearing the hallmark of science and technology. Furthermore, these relations to medicine, and through it to science, technology, and expertise, appear to be the *prototype of a relation to social reality that more often than not is conflictive.*

Two consequences flow from this fact: firstly, health and illness are no longer merely the individual's affair. They have become the centre of debates and collective movements in which can be felt the impact and influence of the representations that we have analyzed together with their evolution.

Secondly, one of the basic things at stake in these collective phenomena is the very existence of the lay discourse and above all, *whether it has any right to discuss or relevance in discussing biological facts*. The conflicts and movements taking shape today in various forms around health, illness, and the body are aimed at making people recognize the existence of these conceptions, these discourses, this non-medical culture of bodily phenomena. These representations, which are somehow all the more conscious of themselves, of their specificity and value, for having been threatened by an encroaching medical discourse, wish to assert themselves as a legitimate collective discourse.

There are a number of examples of the debates and movements growing up around these problems in which the sociologist sees, in the very dynamism of social life with the clash between competing representations, the questions and disputes for which health and illness are today the bases. Some of them arise from institutions and knowledge which have come into competition within the field of medicine. Thus the development in the United States of a new discipline, "bioethics", which began to grow into a separate discipline in the late 1960s and which involves not only physicians and biologists but also philosophers, sociologists, theologians and lawyers,[27] highlights how illness and medicine are now part of a series of dilemmas expressing our ambiguous relationship with scientific and social change. Greater knowledge and a wider range of surgical interventions have given us better control over the body but they have also made us more dissatisfied with its limitations, more intolerant of the uncertainty and danger still surrounding it, and more conscious of the risks that this surgery entails. Bioethics deals with this question of the *risks* entailed in surgery and in medical and biological experimentation, and the concomitant *social and moral choices*. Initially, research concentrated on "patients' rights", the problems of the restricted availability of rare therapies and hence that of choosing the patients to receive them, the problem of defining life and death and the possibility of regulating them by means of abortion and euthanasia. Today bioethical thought has broadened to include medical and biological experimentation, whether by psychosurgery or behaviour therapy, and in particular, genetic experimentation.

In France, problems such as these have only recently been raised, but in the United States, bioethics has taken firm root. Courses in bioethics are offered in an increasing number of American universities as part of the core curriculum in medicine. Hospitals have ethics committees. Several large foundations and institutions[28] are devoted to the study of these problems, colloquiums and publications abound. This broadening probably represents less the flourishing of a social movement than the development of a new university discipline. It is specialists from other academic fields who are moving into medicine with a different "professional" representation and are attempting to dominate, so to speak, medical representations. We might also note that many physicians, particularly researchers and senior hospital physicians, quite willingly accept a dialogue with other specialists that in fact reinforces a positive self-image centred on the importance and the dramatic nature of their responsibilities. A further question arises as to whether it is not in part misguided to try and state in ethical terms problems that are largely predetermined by economic and social factors.

Nevertheless, we cannot but be sensitive to the questions taking shape here and which show how some of the fundamental uncertainties in our relationship with society are projected onto the development of medicine and biology. People are acutely aware of the difficult problems that the development of medical technology and biological experimentation raise for the individual and society, and are unwilling to accept the risks, the possibility of damaging accidents which we can sometimes not even foresee. These notions of "risk",[29] "chance", and "error", found everywhere today in the discourse on illness, are thus not connected with any fatalistic view, but with the ideas of responsibility and treatment. The desire for control grows even stronger when confronted with an unbearable unpredictability, vaguely bound up with the feeling that our all-powerfulness is reprehensible, a transgression of the laws of nature. It is also striking that the notion of risk is being enlarged almost indefinitely. People are now publishing what could be called "second generation" articles. The first articles dealt with the need to control risks; the most recent look at the secondary risks arising from that very control.[30]

But these attempts at control take the form of a return to traditional moral thought. There is a belief that these problems can at least be tackled, if not solved, by building or reconstructing an ethic that is specific to the field but fairly traditional in its principles, and which might possibly be embodied in legislation. The rule must address the questions of transgression, risk, and danger. This is an unprecedented step, but owing to that very fact, the discourse on bioethics is arousing an interest that transcends academic circles. First evidence of this could be found, for example, in the enormous success of certain books on death, such as the book by Elisabeth Kubler-Ross,[31] which sold several million copies within a few years, or the large number of trials and the heated debates over euthanasia, organ donation, unorthodox therapies, etc. The heros of these "causes celebres", the Karen Quinlan case has been well publicized in Europe but there are many others besides,[32] are seen as truly exemplary figures around whom people are seeking to build the new ethic.

There is, however, another facet of the challenging of social reality through medicine, and that is movements of patients and health care users themselves. These movements are based on the idea of an *independent "taking in charge" of his condition* by the patient himself, and the affirmation of the *value of the lay conception, of its right to assert itself* alongside, and possibly in opposition to, medical knowledge. These representations are usually embodied in group movements and practices, patients' associations, "self-care" or "self-help" groups, "health shops", etc. All of them challenge medical technology and knowledge, but what is more, they reject dependence on a physician. The "professional" no longer has the right to single-handedly decide and impose on the patient his own view of illness.

These movements can take very different forms, however. There are the chronically ill, first of all, diabetics,[33] for example, or kidney patients who treat themselves through home dialysis. In these cases, the relationship with the physician's knowledge and practice is that of a *negotiation* that may involve some co-operation. With these lengthy, irreversible ailments for which the patient is hospitalized only for short periods and where he must maintain a social existence, it is often the physician who first feels the need to let the patient share in a certain amount of medical information and to delegate to him certain aspects of his treatment. Taking over from there, however, the patient usually assembles, through contact with others in "patients' groups", a body of specific knowledge based on day-to-day observation and his perception, infinitely more detailed than the doctor's can possibly be, of the biological, psychological and social interactions in his daily life. In some cases, the patient eventually masters medical techniques, haemodialysis, for example, as well as or even better than the professionals, as far as he is concerned. But this mastery of knowledge and technology, this new relationship with science and the professional's power, goes beyond control (no matter how great that control may be) over the individual's biological fate, beyond the victory over his somatic illness.[34] These things have symbolic value: the "new patient", the "self-treating patient", the patient with a "self-care illness", is a new figure in our culture. A patient who is no longer passive, a user who has mastered use, he breaks with one of the central dichotomies of our societies: the often-criticized dichotomy between those who know and impose their knowledge, and those who can only submit to it. He has thus been able, through his body, to establish a new relationship with social reality.

The other aspect of some of these groups is that they call into question and reject medicine. Extreme examples can be found in certain associations of cancer patients.[35] Faced with the failures and limitations of current therapies and the constraints they impose, patients join together, at first to try and ease their solitude and for mutual emotional support: they "learn to be sick" and later, perhaps, together they try to accept the idea of death. But they also want to try and evaluate what modern medicine has to offer them and, finally, to find "other pathways" aside from medical techniques, which they feel to be both ineffective and mutilating.

We can see in these groups the evolution of the collective conceptions of illness that we have analyzed. The same antitheses are at work here, but they have taken on a new meaning. The conception of illness asserting itself here marks the advent of a neo-hippocratic theory according to which the individual's resistance, his "will to recover", his fundamental "healthiness", are the essential weapons, a "medicine in itself"[36] against an illness which always originates in society's aggression but which is compounded by medical treatment. "Soft" therapies which act on the "area", strengthening "resistance" are, on the other hand, equated with "nature" and man's fundamental "healthiness". Herein, it is believed, lies true efficacity, whereas medicine, not only powerless but actually destructive, is simply the counterpart of a harmful society felt to be at the origin of illness. The patient is fighting a battle on three fronts: against illness, against medicine, and against a society which legitimates, and expresses itself through, medicine. With his body suffering, he also claims the right to the social deviance of refusing medical care, and it is through this deviance alone that he hopes to recover.[37]

Whether they opt for negotiations or take a rigid stance of rebellion and rejection, all of these movements share a particular way of *articulating the individual and the collective*. We are dealing with groups which are explicitly asserting the collective dimension of their action. The participants are stating that they cannot take charge of their illness independently without the mutual support of the group members and the exchange of information and experience leading to the elaboration of collective knowledge distinct from the knowledge of the physician. But the stakes are still the individual's: to overcome *my* illness, regain *my* health. These groups express, paradoxically, a collective focus (even, at times, an introversion) on the individual. In fact, this contradiction is another of their assertions. Groups of ill persons often claim to have a political purpose, but they link that purpose to the individual dimension of their activity. It is "because it is individual", they say, "that it is political."[38]

It can of course be argued that these are little more than marginal, fragmented, tenuous movements whose importance should not be overestimated. It is true that "patients' groups" or "health shops", for instance, are often small undertakings, isolated, short-lived, and easily ended. But they are part of a greater whole: ecology groups and anti-science movements share some of their ideas, and a whole new type of militancy[39] is challenging society today through aspects of the individual's everyday life. The activity of these groups must also be seen in the context of the new body awareness[40] that exists today, and of the growing symbolic importance of the notion of health.[41] Health, body, and nature are seen as our fundamental assets, both individual and collective, threatened by social development. The movements related to them, the struggles to defend them against "alienating" and "aggressive" society, are perhaps not far distant from the social struggles of the past. Health is also becoming a normative super-category, with multiple meanings and a multi-dimensional field of action:[42] health is in everything, and everything is in health. It has been said that health is one of the new synonyms for happiness.

These movements are not without ambiguity, however. If health becomes a supreme value, then not being healthy may become a serious fault. The new value being attached to health, like the claims for self-care of biological illness, imply a potential "victim blaming" which must not be underestimated. They could also open the way to a standardizing health ideology. Certainly, the claim of individuality found in all the movements is undoubtedly the best defence against the threat of such an ideology which, in France at least, is still a weak one, but it too has its dangers. The desire for individual responsibility is in line with the public discourse, now criticizing the rising cost of health care. "Your health is your business" could signify a retreat from social consciousness and public health care. Here again, the management of biological illness lies at the centre of the contradictions between the individual and the social.

NOTES

1. Quoted by G. Rosen in "The evolution of medicine", H.E. Freeman, S. Levine and L.G. Reeder, eds., *Handbook of Medical Sociology*, 3rd ed., Englewood Cliffs, N.J., Prentice Hall, 1979, pp. 23-50.
2. For example: A.B. Hollingshead and F.C. Redlich, *Social Class and Mental Illness*, New York, J. Wiley, 1958.
3. Cf. A. Antonovsky, "Breakdown: a needed fourth step in the conceptual armamentarium of modern medicine", *Social Science and Medicine*, VI, 1972, pp. 537-544.
4. Cf. for example the following collections: H.E. Freeman, S. Levine and L.G. Reeder, eds., *Handbook of Medical Sociology*, op. cit.; E. Gartly Jaco, ed., *Patients, Physicians and Illness*, New York, The Free Press, 1958, 3rd ed. 1978; D. Mechanic, ed., *Medical Sociology*, New York, The Free Press, 1968, 2nd ed., 1978. See in French: C. Herzlich, ed., *Médecine, maladie et société*, Paris, Mouton, 1970.
5. T. Parsons, "Social structure and dynamic process: the case of modern medical practice." *In: The Social System*. The Free Press 1951 ch x pp. 428–480 Cf. also: T. Parsons and R.C. Fox, "Illness, therapy and the modern urban family", *Journal of Social Issues*, VIII, 1952, pp. 31-44.
6. D. Mechanic, "The concept of illness behaviour", *Journal of Chronic Diseases*, XV, 1962, pp. 189-194.
7. Cf. for example: D. Apple, "How laymen define illness", *Journal of Health and Human Behaviour*, I, 1960, pp. 219-225, and B. Baumann, "Diversities in conceptions of health and physical fitness", *Journal of Health and Human Behaviour*, II, 1961, pp. 39-46.
8. Cf. for example the collection by L. Bozzini and M. Renaud, *Médecine et société: les années 80*, Montréal, Editions coopératives Albert Saint Martin, coll. "Recherches et documents", 1981.
9. See Eliot Freidson's formulation in *Profession of Medicine: a Sociology of Applied Knowledge*, New York, Dodd and Mead, 1970, part III, "The social construction of illness".
10. This is an application of P.G. Berger and T. Luckmann's theory, *The Social Construction of Reality, a Treatise in the Sociology of Knowledge*, New York, Doubleday, 1966.

11. Cf. E. Freidson, "Client's control and medical practice" *American Journal of Sociology*, 1960, 65 pp. 374–382.
12. S.Y. Fagerhaugh and A. Strauss, *Politics of Pain Management*, Menlo Park, Cal., Addison Wesley, 1977.
13. For example: T. Scheff, *Being Mentally Ill*, Chicago, Aldine, 1966.
14. For example: J. Roth, "Ritual and magic in the control of contagion", *American Sociological Review*, XXII, 1957, pp. 310-314; R.C. Fox, *Experiment Perilous: Physicians and Patients Facing the Unknown*, New York, The Free Press, 1959; Tina Posner, "Magical elements in orthodox medicine", in R. Dingwall et al., eds., *Health Care and Health Knowledge*, London, Croom Helm, 1977.
15. I. Baszanger, *Des généralistes en particulier: une approche biographique des processus de socialisation professionnelle* (PhD thesis, EHESS, 1979).
16. This term still appears occasionally in French medical literature.
17. Cf. T.J. Scheff, "Decision rules, types of error and their consequences in medical diagnosis", *Behavioural Science*, 1963, 8, pp. 97–107.
18. Many examples of this could be given: it is known that the black plague in the Middle Ages killed over one quarter of the population of Europe. Napoleon was said to have been defeated first of all by General Typhus, etc.
19. Cf. M.R. Bury and P.H.N. Wood, "Problems of communication in chronic illness", *International Rehabilitation Medicine* (Basel), I, 1979, pp. 130-134.
20. Susan Sontag, *Illness as Metaphor*, New York, Farrar, Strauss and Giroux, 1977.
21. Marc Augé, *Théorie des pouvoirs et idéologie: étude de cas en Côte d'Ivoire*, Paris, Hermann, coll. avoir, 1975.
22. C. Herzlich, *Santé et maladie: analyse d'une réprésentation sociale*, Paris, Mouton, 1969, English translation: *Health and Illness, a Social Psychological Analysis*. Academic Press, 1973.
23. The term "psychosomatic" was not frequently used in the 1960s. It is common usage today.
24. This can be contrasted to the fact that some workers, particularly miners, were keenly aware of it in the 19th century. In 1848, during an enquiry into labour in the National Assembly, a miner testified that unless the living and working conditions of miners were improved, "most workers would soon be unfit to work beyond the age of 35 or 45." He added: "It is recognized that the average life expectancy of miners is no more than 38 or 40 years." Quoted by R. Trempe, "Les luttes des ouvriers mineurs français pour la création des caisses de retraite au XIXe siècle", speech at the colloquium on "Développement et effets sociaux des politiques de la vieillesse dans les pays industrialisés". In Jn A.M. Guillemand, Old Age and the Welfare State, Russel Sage, 1984. It should be further noted that in the 1970s there was renewed awareness of the connection between work and health. Cf., for example, the Pennaroya Enterprises union dispute between 1972 and 1975.
25. Since this chapter was written, the situation has been deeply transformed by the AIDS epidemic.

26. For example: A. D'Houtaud, "Les représentations de la sante", *Revue inter-nationale d'éducation pour la santé*, XIX, 2, 1976, pp. 99-118; 3, pp. 173-190.
27. For an analysis of the development of bioethics, see R.C. Fox, "Ethical and existential developments in contemporaneous American medicine: their implications for culture and society", *Health and Society*, LI, 1974, pp. 445-583.
28. In particular The Institute of Society, Ethics and the Life Sciences in Hastings on Hudson (State of New York) and the Joseph and Rose Kennedy Institute of Georgetown University in Washington.
29. Cf. in a different sphere the many discussions of "risk factors" in the onset of illness.
30. Cf. D.L. Bazelon, "Risk and responsibility", *Science* (Washington), CCV, 1979, pp. 277-280.
31. E. Kübler-Ross, *On Death and Dying*, London, Collier-MacMillan, 1969.
32. Cf. on this point the article by Renee C. Fox, "The evolution of medical uncertainty", *Health and Science*, LVIII, 1980, pp. 1-47.
33. A Hervouet, *Le diabète insulino-dépendent: deux idéologies médicales, deux modalités therapeutiques, deux attitudes du malade* (DEA thesis, EHESS, 1979, 131 typed pp.)
34. The failures also show, *a contrario*, that the body is not the only thing at stake. In their book *The Courage to Fail* (op. cit.) R. Fox and J. Swazey examine at length the case of a young working-class American Indian, Ernie Crowfeather, who had irreversible kidney disease in both kidneys and was treated by hemodialysis thanks to financial aid from the Indian community. The young man courted death both through his body --he provoked a number of incidents and relapses --and through his behaviour: he never managed to adapt to home dialysis, missed treatment sessions, ran away from the hospital and ended up dying. But his quasi-suicide expresses his revolt against a situation in which biological illness, subjection to a machine, dependency on health care practitioners and gratefulness to the donors were constantly intermingled and could lead to only one thing: the impossibility of an independent life and the need for annihilation.
35. Cf. on this subject the special issue of *Autrement* (No. 26, Sept. 1980): *La santé à bras-le-corps*. It should be noted that not all associations of cancer patients adhere to these conceptions.
36. N. Cousins, "*Anatomy of an Illness as perceived by the Patient: Reflections on Healing and Regeneration*" New York, W.W. Norton, 1979.
37. All of these themes appear in a trial that created a sensation in the United States a few years ago. A group of doctors brought an action against the parents of Chad Greed, a 2-year-old boy with leukemia, requesting that the child be taken out of the custody of the parents, who had stopped his chemotherapy treatment to take him to Mexico to put him on a vegetarian diet together with injections of laetril, a drug that was not accepted by the medical profession. The question at issue in the trial was whether parents had a right to refuse medical treatment in favour of "alternative" therapy, and to opt for what they called a "good life" (without the side effects of chemotherapy) as opposed to a "long life" for their child. Cf. R.C. Fox, "The evolution of medical uncertainty", op. cit.

38. Cf., for example, G. Briche, "Au carrefour du solitaire et du politique", in *La santé à bras-le-corps*, op. cit., pp. 11-20.

39. This new militancy has been seen as typical of a "new middle class", cf. for example M. Dagnaud and D. Mehl, *La troisième classe* (Paris, Centre d'études des mouvements sociaux, March 1981, 33 typed pp.)

40. Cf. D. Jodelet et al., *Système de représentation du corps et groupes sociaux* (Research report, EHESS, 1980, 271 typed pp.)

41. Cf. J. Pierret's article in this volume.

42. R. Crawford, "Healthism and the medicalization of everyday life", *International Journal of Health Services*, X, 1980, pp. 365-388.

Chapter 6

THE SOCIAL MEANINGS OF HEALTH: PARIS, THE ESSONNE, THE HERAULT

J. Pierret

These past years have been marked by the emergence of health as a core concept in the field of medicine and in society as a whole. Such a situation cannot but be of interest to sociologists insofar as the relationship between health and illness, normality and pathology is "socially formed and is a key to a society's global system of interpretations, beliefs and values."[1] If we start from the fact that technico-scientific medicine was built up and developed on the basis of illness, it would seem legitimate to examine the significance of this swing in interest towards health. There is in fact, a new distinction in real life between what is and what is not illness which both fulfils a certain number of social, political and economic functions and leads to the interpretation of medicine itself and its relationship with society. It is a question then of examining in what context and form bio-medical science has been led to question its epistemological assumptions. The whole community is affected by the way medical science constructs its aims and is concerned by its changes in perspective. The various social groups organise all their social and symbolic behaviour coherently into systems of interpretations and we understand health as providing a way of approach to these various productions. Laymen have several ways of speaking about health because for them the word health implies at one and the same time illness and medicine, work, education and family and behind these different conceptions of health can be understood the meaning that individuals give to their social behaviour and habits.

I MEDICINE: BETWEEN ILLNESS AND HEALTH

Modern medicine acquired its legitimacy as a science by evolving around a physico-chemical approach to the illness it witnessed in the body of the individual. Illness, the body, the individual and science are the pillars of technico-scientific medicine. By studying various symptoms in the body in order to identify them, bring them together into larger groups and identify their mechanisms and discover their causes and aetiology, medicine created its own subject, illness. As Jean Clavreul[2] suggested, the medical discourse is a discourse on illness and not on the sick man, "the patient's role is simply to provide information on the state of the ailing body." In developing its corpus of knowledge, its technical means of research and its methods of therapeutical intervention with illness at the centre, technico-scientific medicine failed to consider the human being as a bio-psycho-social entity. Moreover, this illness-subject constructed by bio-medicine has gradually been imposed as a natural subject. In this process, it was forgotten that illness is not a subject in itself but is one particular way of drawing a distinction in society at a given moment between normality and pathology, as Georges Canguilhem had already showed in 1943 in his thesis for his degree in medicine, "Normality and Pathology".[3] Lastly, modern medicine's logical rational approach to medicine made it difficult to conceive of any other approach and obscured the social dimension, i.e. the individual and social meaning of illness.

When, at certain times in the course of its history, medicine raised the question of its social dimension, it did so mainly in terms of social causality and aetiology, forgetting that illness is always a part of a society to which it refers us and about which it reveals something. In particular, the 19th century saw the development of a wide-ranging movement in medical topography and geography, more generally known as "hygienism". Medicine disposed of scant means to improve knowledge and treatment. Although the anatomic-clinical method was appearing on the scene, it had not yet, as Michel Foucault[4] shows, transformed hospitals from simple places of shelter into places for producing medicine nor had it infiltrated medical practice to convert it into a rigorous and rational way to approach illness. Medicine was powerless to check epidemics which continued to wipe out whole communities. This became even more apparent as nascent industrialisation had gathered the manpower it needed into workshops and urban centres, a concentration in the workplace and in cities, with the latter being what most attracted the attention of the hygienist movement, as can be seen from the reports of the "Conseils de salubrite", set up in 1802. The task of these councils, originally made up of chemists but from 1832 onwards including doctors, engineers and architects, was to inform the government on all aspects of public health and hygiene. Minutely detailed reports were drawn up about urban areas, villages, workshops and living quarters with particular attention to air and light. "It is particularly under this twofold aspect that the building of houses and the laying out of roads, villages and cities should be considered of the utmost importance for public health (...) it is there that the germs of innumerable illnesses and the causes of premature death are to be found", as we can read in the 1824 report, quoted by Roger H. Guerrand.[5] Throughout France, monographs on the subject have facilitated the compilation of statistics on living and working conditions and their relations to certain illnesses.

Laws were even passed such as the 1850 Law on unhealthy housing or the 1874 law governing child labour. This interest in the social aetiology of illness and the health of the nation was, however, only shown by a section of the medical profession, those who were members of the "Conseils de salubrite" and later of the "Conseils d'hygiene publique" whose views were published in the "Annales d'hygiene publique et de medicine legale" and who were in contact with the public authorities and the Government. But in the last quarter of the nineteenth century, by singling out germs as the cause of illness, the "Pasteur Revolution" was to provide one and only one explanation for illness and social factors were relegated to the background. The "hygienist" movement now had a scientific rationale: germs are everywhere. However, theirs was not the only approach. There were also the various approaches of the nineteenth century philanthropic movement. This liberal movement believing in free enterprise and private property and including part of the *bourgeois* business class and the Catholic world, sought to maintain the existing social order by providing medical assistance (dispensaries, home visits). Upholding the values of the family and private property, they proposed that the working class model itself on the *bourgeoisie* and emulate its ethics such as order, regularity, discipline and providence", as Pierre Leroy-Beaulieu wrote in 1872 in *La question ouvriere au XIXe siecle.*[6] Medicine was of course one of the instruments for introducing moral principles to the working class.

Medicine imposed its views on personal hygiene and health through child care and child upbringing and through compulsory schooling where it was the task of primary school teachers to introduce hygiene as one of the pillars of lay morality. Supported by certain elements of the bourgeoisie close to the Radicals, the "hygienist" movement wanted to use political power to influence people's lives in an attempt to ward off the possible destruction of society as a result of the physical and moral depravation of the population. The result was that some of them took local or national political office. Above all, they strove to improve the water supply, the drainage system and sanitation in the towns. In the course of their endeavours, they generally came up against one basic problem: the dire poverty of the lower classes; a pathogenic poverty which nurtured immorality, vice, debauchery and its own moral code.[7] The precepts of wisdom, moderation, sobriety and the happy medium were introduced on a large scale and used in the battle against the social ills of the time: tuberculosis, venereal diseases and alcoholism. The war against microbes gradually became a war against germ carriers.

Since it was unsuccessful in curing and effectively combatting epidemics and social ills, one section of the medical profession devoted its energy to hygiene and, concentrating on the social environment, studied the latter's relation to illness. It was in the very places that they undertook their research (towns, workshops, dwellings) and through the very solutions they proposed, that they came face to face with the basic problem of dire poverty. Poverty and vice then were two aspects of the same reality, the working class. In Dr. Leon Boyer's words in 1868, "the hygienist was imposed as a teacher of moral conduct"[8] and an attempt was made to inculcate in this dangerous class a moral code based on cleanliness, moderation and virtue.

Starting in the late nineteenth century organicist and curative medicine was developed, seeking its knowledge in the sick body, due to the contributions of bacteriology and physiology and insuring that it had the means to undertake research and therapy. Thenceforth, illness became the focus of medical reflection and progress. In the best Pasteurian tradition, illness seemed unpredictable and usually caused by a foreign pathogenic element which, if identified and isolated, could be treated and the individual restored to his former state. The aim was to compensate for the unpredictability of illness by improving the medical infrastructure and making medical care and doctors more readily available. Since illness could not be prevented, it would have to be cured. From this viewpoint, it is illness that makes people conscious of health as a possession lost and then found again through healing. Health, however, was not actually experienced, it could only be measured in relation to illness and as Leriche says, "health is life in the silence of the body's organs". So the medical profession strove to overcome illness and even to eliminate it so as to restore the patient to that normal and healthy state which is good health; a state that it knew very little about although it was responsible for its recovery. So paradoxically health can be defined as the absence of illness and as the summum of positiveness or even, in the broader definition of the World Health Organization, as "a state of total physical, mental and social well-being". It would not be doing justice to the notion of health to reduce it to a mere state especially as this would tend to overlook the fact that it serves to pose the relationship between normality and pathology. This relationship is essentially social because of its historical and cultural context but especially because it holds the key to understanding a particular type of social organization and can reveal something about it.

However, at the peak of technico-scientific medicine when it had proved its worth towards its subject, illness, a certain interest in health reemerged. V. Navarro[9] rightly emphasized the fact that it was not thanks to, but rather in spite of, the medical profession that the definition of health and medical services changed. In fact, the redefinition of values follows a certain social logic that cannot be reduced simply to a professional logic but implies taking account of all the interests involved. It was precisely because the '70s raised a series of social and political questions about technological and hyper-specialized medicine that changes appear on the horizon. Medicine in the sense of a body of professionals with sole power to intervene in illness and health was contested. It was contested from without by a new train of thought which denounced the hold that doctors had over "the sick body", dispossessing the individual. The feminist and self-care movement in the United States and the Mouvement pour la Liberte de l'Avortement et Contraception (MLAC) in France were the major exponents of this new way of thinking. By publishing "Medical Nemesis" in 1975, Ivan Illich popularized a debate on the limits of medicine and its effectiveness, which until then had been limited to academic circles and fostered by R.J. Carlson, J. Powles and A. Cochrane.[10] The results of a new discipline, epidemiology, helped change traditional ideas on medicine. The idea that illness could be caused by one exogenous factor was abandoned and there was increasing talk of a more multi-causal and reticular approach. In this way, the illness-recovery schema was gradually replaced by an illness-stabilization type of schema. Furthermore, mortality and morbidity patterns also changed. The importance of infectious diseases declined and there was a corresponding increase in the incidence of degenerative pathologies, ailments involving complex immunity processes, and violent deaths. These illnesses, which have even been called the "illnesses of civilization" can mainly be attributed to environment and lifestyle. The scientific community widely disseminates this view of things and public opinion becomes increasingly aware of topics such as air pollution, water contamination, pesticides, food colourings and additives, safety in the workplace, etc., which medicine is powerless to contain. Then the question of medicine's efficiency is raised, in view of the substantial increase in health costs, and of its efficacy in view of the regression and even disappearance of a certain number of illnesses prior to the advent of technico-scientific medicine and hence independently of its action. Hence in France there was talk at the time of the VIIth Plan of "entering into a phase of diminishing returns from the point of view of medical efficacity".[11]

Health then came to the fore. Whereas it used to provide justification for all action taken by curative medicine, in recent years it has come to play a prominent role in its own right. It is defined as "the state of health of the nation" ascertained through an examination of factors such as life expectancy, causes of death and morbidity. The economic aspect of health can no longer be ignored especially since the State is involved in financing medical costs. Already in 1973, the Canadians had put forward the idea of "a health field concept" based on four main elements: human biology, the environment, lifestyle, and the health care system.[12] According to this idea, health care is not confined merely to curative treatment and its new objects are to be treated in a less pragmatic way, similar to the way that medicine treats illness, that is, on the basis of scientific research based on new concepts, risk factors assessed according to the individual's habits and socio-economic environment. This "health field concept" was adopted by French planners and figured with clear explanations in the report on the VII Plan.[13] Health was presented as a multiform concept involving the health care system but also implying that the environment (that is, all elements outside the body over which it has no control) must be taken into account as must people's living conditions and way of life. Health was seen as a collective patrimony to be protected and reinforced by taking the necessary steps. Finally, health was everyman's duty to himself and society, each of us being to a large extent answerable for his own health. This responsibility must be accepted once people have been encouraged and taught how to do so by an appropriate health education.

That was why until the 1960s, the unforeseeable nature of illness necessitated the development of the medical infrastructure because in the absence of any means of prevention, cure was the only solution. "The right to health" used to mean that everybody should have equal access to medical services. Today it has a different meaning. It means giving each person a sense of responsibility for his own health and to this end each one has to adopt a code of rational behaviour to help him to face up to the pathogenic effects of his lifestyle. For in the health sector, condemning a way of life does not imply calling the whole economic and social structure into question but rather developing personal strategies to cope with it. Each citizen must be responsible for his own health and act in such a manner as to exclude unhealthy behaviour. In 1972, V. Fuchs wrote: "The link between individual behaviour and a large number of health problems has become more and more obvious. In the absence of major discoveries in medical science, the greatest possibilities for improving health lie in individuals changing their attitudes, in what they do or do not do for themselves."[14] Marc Renaud[15] summed this up with the following formula: "Whereas previously 'the right to health' referred to the principle that people 'had the right to be ill and receive adequate treatment,' now all of a sudden people have the 'duty to be healthy.'"

The emergence of health as a basic value means that it is no longer simply a means to an end but an end in itself. Health becomes the very definition of life and medical science is now able to indicate the way to live, as I.K. Zola[16] points out. G. Canguilheim[17] had emphasized the fact that the concept of normality and health contains a twofold reference. One is a "descriptive" reference which considers abnormal any change in the individual's normal self (i.e., a certain aptitude to face up to social and biological reality) perceived by himself or by an outsider. The second is a "normative" reference which makes it possible to discover peculiarities or anomalies in an individual by comparing him with what we know of others. With regard to the species in general, norms are necessary to be able to recognize anomalies. Today, it is as though the emphasis put on health has sacrificed its descriptive dimension and its reference to illness to its normative dimension. It would seem that the problem is no longer one of remedying a dysfunction and eliminating the illness but rather of proposing a new lifestyle and encouraging behaviour which is favourable to good health. With health the norm, people need to be taught to manage their lives as though it was life that needed to be cured.[18] Moreover, this new norm tends to focus on "victim blaming",[19] in other words, the plea for personal responsibility is based on the idea of individual freedom and independence from social constraints. These constraints are considered as one ubiquitous entity which applies to everyone in the same way regardless of their position. It is understood then that informing each person of the risks he runs implies that he has an obligation to avoid them. And so we pass from the conception of "illness-risk" in terms of a posteriori insurance and guarantee, to a conception of "risk of illness" in terms of a priori cause and responsibility. Moreover, the factors recognized as risk factors are given an aetiological status which is not always proven and thus can often be mistakenly considered the cause of an illness or even the illness itself. Smoking, for example, which is a risk factor for bronchial cancer, becomes a cause of cancer and even an illness in itself. As N. Bensaid[20] writes, "The most that can be said is that a risk factor increases, in varying proportions, our risk of dying and being ill. It does not actually bring it about (in that case, it would be a cause). Eliminating the risk factor does not eliminate the risk. Yet this is what is insinuated by those who inform the public and believed by those who are informed, as though illness, suffering, insanity or death could be avoided instead of simply being part of life."

These changes in the medical field were wrought not only by those in the profession but were influenced by a much wider range of social factors, involving various and even contradictory political and economic interests. In this context of redefining values, it seems appropriate to examine the role that the community as a whole plays or does not play and its attitude towards this process. In other words, medicine presents only *one* particular view of reality as the true one but there are other possible constructions, there are other ways of conceiving the relationship between normality and pathology. And it is these views that the layman has in mind when he talks of health and the way he organizes his social and symbolic practices into a coherent schema of interpretation. Health is a key to understanding the various views and conceptions of the different social classes. Their conceptions unveil a certain philosophy of life or at least a certain meaning given to life.

II THE DIFFERENT DISCURSIVE USES OF HEALTH AND THEIR SOCIAL MEANING

The following analysis is the result of research based on fieldwork carried out on a random sample of over 100 persons, including white and blue collar workers, middle and top management from a typical

Parisian area in the XIIth arrondissement and a housing estate in the Val d'Yerres in the Essonne departement and also including farmers from an area in the Herault department. For the purpose of the research each person underwent a tape-recorded, non-directive interview and filled in a closed questionnaire aimed at discovering their behavioural patterns with regard to health care, housing, work, eating habits, tobacco, alcohol, and physical exercise...[21]

It turned out that asking non-professionals to talk about health was like asking them to talk about their habits in general: about physical habits regarding food and hygiene, social habits relating to work, home life and environment or even the children's upbringing. For talking about health is tantamount to talking about life. This meant putting them in a position to explore the whole social spectrum and question their relationship with it. The analysis went on from there to attempt to bring out the different ways to give a meaning to the notion of health and vice versa. People's conception of health provides a key to the meaning that they give to their behaviour and their social habits. What is more, dealing with time, the body, space and safety in a corpus on health presupposes that a particular discourse is related to all other possible discourses and that habits are not independent of other habits. So, far from narrowing the discourse, we consider it rather to be a significant aspect of the ideo-logic. Because, as Marc Auge[22] writes: "The major themes of economic, social or political organization are the object of their representations, in the same way as religious organization; or to be more precise, organization and representation are always given together, there cannot be organization without representation... However, there is no discourse without a subject and society is not a subject. Thus, to construct the ideo-logic, we only possess incomplete discourses which insinuate it without completely revealing it. The ideo-logic is not the sum total of all the discourses that the wisest, most experienced of its members could provide on society. It is the basic structure (syntactic logic) for all possible discourses in a given society on that society."

With that in mind, a classification of "forms of health" (to use Claudine Herzlich's[23] expression) has been drawn up. Four forms have been constructed based on the meaning spontaneously given to the notion of health by those interviewed and they constitute relatively coherent ways to establish discourses. Each form of health is developed according to its logic which makes it possible to give meaning to the way of placing each person in society as a whole and develop relationships between nature, body and society. It is nonetheless difficult to give them a sociological interpretation and it would be too early to identify social situations and, *a fortiori*, social groups, favouring the expression of one group or another, even if we can advance the hypothesis of a certain "social predisposition" to each expression. Moreover, the manifesting of life logics underlying these conceptions of health will only be hypothetical insofar as the analysis is not completely finished.

Health is: not being ill ...

Health is most often perceived in relation to illness. This was the case for almost half the people interviewed and constitutes the "health-illness" form, the dominant and most heterogenous form. It is heterogeneous partly because it includes people from all the social classes and it is thus difficult to situate it sociologically. However, it includes an over high proportion of men, Parisians, under-forties, and households with an average to high income. It is also heterogeneous because of its discourse on illness. However, illness is always in the fore and a point of reference either as an experience that the person interviewed has actually lived or as the very definition of health in terms of absence of illness. The fact that some describe their "experience" while others define the notion of health, may be explained by the greater capacity for abstraction of some social categories but for everybody it is illness that has a meaning here. Illness leads to awareness of health as a complex positive state of interrelations between the physical and the psychic. Health is not the yardstick; people become aware of it only when they have lost it.

The ubiquity of illness shapes their whole discourse and gives a particular meaning to the various habits, be they corporeal or social. In this form, the argumentation is based on contrasts and differences: city versus country, today versus yesterday, pathogenic society versus healthy body, inside versus outside.... In fact, the discourse is dominated by the idea that city life implies toxic products, poisons, and other chemical substances that threaten the individual's overall wellbeing. A pathogenic society is responsible for all our ills. The constant reference to illness leads to awareness of the body or rather, of a particular type of body: a partial and compartmentalized object, apprehended mainly in terms of symptoms, organs and functions. Little attention is given to the "play-body", the body as a source of pleasure. When the pleasures of the body are mentioned, it is in relation to special occasions (parties, holidays). In this form, it seems that the clinical approach has infiltrated ideas of the body. The anatomical and physiological body does however assimilate the experiences of each one. The notion of balance always underlies the understanding of all bodily habits, be they related to illness, eating or hygiene. This balance, which is to be maintained or restored, is both an aim and a rule. Moderation is recommended, social and physical habits are characterized by the idea of balance. It is a question of "neither too much nor too little" and of striking the right balance. This could be understood as "a normal life" as in G. Canguilheim's conclusion: "The normal man feels capable of failing his body but lives in the certitude of being able to put off the moment. In the case of illness, the 'normal man' is the one who lives with the assurance that he can, in himself, halt a process which would continue to the bitter end in another. The normal man, if he is to believe and declare himself normal, does not need a foretaste of illness but its mere shadow."[24]

In this form, illness is associated with an organic or psychic, but usually external, dysfunction. It is often integrated into a complex pattern of multiple causes where microbes, climate and heredity are mingled and which is denominated by excesses and lifestyle. The individual is attacked, the body threatened and the balance upset. Illness is due to excess and plenty: we suffer from overwork, oversmoking and overeating..., we are sick of the city, noise and transport. Abuse of tobacco, alcohol and certain foodstuffs is pathogenic, deteriorates the body and upsets the balances. So, we should drink in moderation and eat in moderation, especially fats. The notions of poisons, toxic substances, are associated with tobacco, alcohol and certain foodstuffs because of production conditions and the economic interests at stake, preventing people eating a healthy, natural diet.... It should be noticed that medicines are also considered synonymous with toxicity, if taken in large doses. Thus, moderation is essential and excesses should be remedied by having a personal prescription for each one: drinking water to rid the body of toxic substances after heavy drinking, cycling to get rusty joints back in working order, fresh country air to rid the lungs of petrol fumes. These are the "ploys" used by those in the "health-illness" group. They are empirical methods, acquired through experience that they have no intention of generalizing or recommending to others. Each person must get to know himself and find out what is best for him. This is true only to the extent that maintaining a balance does not mean living a rational life. On the contrary, there are those who believe "you should know how to enjoy yourself and even have a drink too many and go out on the town with your pals now and then." The pleasures of the body are associated with leisure time and hence, with an exceptional situation, and so, in this respect, are considered normal. It is by transgressing the rules that they come to recognize the value of balanced living, in the same way as illness makes them appreciate the importance of health. This calls to mind the advice given by the Salerno school in the 11th century:[25]

"Art wards off illnesses, better than it can cure them,
Air, rest and sleep, pleasure and food,
If taken in moderation, keep man in good health,

Abuse of them turns these pure ingredients into poison
Which ravages the body and disturbs the mind."

Françoise Loux highlighted the fact that advice in late 19th century proverbs lays great emphasis on moderation and that these proverbs outline a theory of respect for the universe's equilibrium. Moderation in everything means running one's life as though one only had a finite amount of energy and leading a calm, orderly life. So it is order which is the central theme of the Salernitan precepts, proverbs and treatises on how to live.

Underlying the ideas behind this form of health are the notions of cycle, rhythm and natural history as though time was acting as a unifying agent. The logic behind this discourse may be that of "the order of things". It is nonetheless not a discourse on determinism, nor even fatality, but one on normality. Working and professional life is seen in this light. There is talk of professional life and work experience rather than of Work as an abstract notion. Aware of being caught up in a system where work is the dominant feature, these categories recognize both the alienation and guarantee it represents. This ambiguity is borne out by their own experience and no way out can be envisaged. Their detailed descriptions of working conditions, the working day prolonged by commuting time, and the pace dictated by the machines' rhythm all add up to a criticism of work. This alienating occupation is unavoidable owing to the general employment situation and the amount of unemployment. It is also pathogenic, exposing the worker to fatigue, stress, overwork and causing accidents and illness. However, although work is subject to serious criticism, it is not rejected, it is not one of the terms of an alternative. It is work itself which is attacked, the time it occupies is lost forever. There is the problem of finding time for living which cannot, as suggested by other people interviewed, be reduced to a question of organizing one's time. But although work is alienating and pathogenic, it is also a guarantee. It provides a means of existence and ensures social benefits and cover. This leads to a certain esteem for work, considered indispensable to the extent that "work means health" but it is not so much a matter of work being felt as something positive as of "not working" being rejected because it opens the path to idleness, the "father of all evils", or to being a social outcast or even in some cases to delinquency. Some people even go so far as to criticize and describe as ill a society that does not ensure its basic social function, i.e., "work for all" with the result that its members are exposed to insecurity and illness. It could be said that in this form, work is a factor of physical, moral and social wellbeing. This does not mean that it is sacred and redeeming. Recognizing its importance is based on a critical analysis of professional working life at its most daily and down-to-earth. To a certain extent, it is an analysis on a debate on "social relations".

Those in this form contemplate different habits in the light of their own experience within a social system from which there is no escape. It seems unnecessary in such circumstances to suggest the adoption of a set of permanent rules on how to live or even a reorganization of their daily lives. The notions of balance and natural cycle, in the way that they take account of a certain link with time, shed light on some aspects of this form of health. It is in particular, the meaning of what is said about illness. They seem to consider it as something that happens suddenly and without warning. "Illness takes a grip on you, suddenly, out of the blue" and even if an explanation is found, it is always a posteriori. One should always be prepared because if illness happens unexpectedly, treatment is required. This should be encouraged by better medical coverage and more doctors. The fact is that even if illness cannot be foreseen, it is nevertheless closely entrenched in time in which it takes root to search for origins, explanations and a meaning. It reaches forward in time because illness is a process with its own cycles to complete and stages to go through. It can be benign, commonplace, or serious. It can last, get worse and cause complications. It is time which intervenes in the interpretation of the symptoms and the nature of the trouble and decides whether or not to wait before consulting a doctor. Here the expression "normal illness" is used to describe routine troubles such as colds and influenza and children's diseases which are part of the life cycle. Farmers who share this view clearly express the idea of natural illness in that they do not see human and animal illness (illness, nature and work) as separate things but rather as part of the same whole. Waiting for an illness to pass is like waiting for the rain to stop or a ewe to give birth. By schematizing this viewpoint, we can say that illness is considered part of life, and that health means being able to fall ill and recover. Thus prevention, often seen as prediction, is looked upon with a certain amount of suspicion because there is no need to know, there will be time enough when the illness happens. Doctor Bensaid also speaks of this confusion between prevention and prediction and adds "Medicine is obviously not alone in wishing to see into the future, so that once foreseen, it could brought under control. This belief or hope gives rise to a dual question: is the determining factor the predictable or the unpredictable aspect and secondly, is it desirable, reassuring, beneficial or necessary to predict?"[26] Referring to a recent study, carried out by M. Blaxter and E. Paterson in Aberdeen, on two generations of lower class women, R. Illsley[27] established a link between a certain scepticism and even fatalism with respect to prevention, and the fact of not giving health a positive meaning.

In this health type, where sickness is the yardstick, physical and social habits are woven around the relationship between normal and patho-logical. It is because our individual and social experience of excesses, abuses and transgressions can only be exceptional that we become aware of a norm. This idea is reiterated by N. Bensaid when he says, "The doctor should recognize the difference between enjoying life and valuing life. It is a matter of experience, the less meaning and interest life holds the more we value it. Those for whom life is an adventure risk it willingly. Conversely, for those who take it for what it is, it becomes their sole possession with its own intrinsic value and they cannot bear the thought of losing it."[28] All personal and collective habits are generally part of the social system or, to be more precise, the system of production. The social system is imposed on everybody but there must be respect for its order and balance because each event has its own rhythm and develops according to a "natural cycle". Time past cannot be recovered, even leisure time does not make up for time spent at work. Consumption does not eliminate the alienation imposed by the system of production, it can merely compensate for it, just as medicine provides a remedy in the event of illness.

Health is the most important thing ...

For almost one out of four people interviewed, health was the yardstick. They constitute the "health-instrument" type; for them, health is what is most important in life, good health is their wealth, their capital. Good health means they can do anything, everything is possible, especially work. This group is socially homogeneous and is composed of those in the sample who come from a modest background, large family-low income bracket and with a low level of education, living for the most part in big apartment blocks in the Paris region as well as of half the farmers interviewed. They represent the survival of the idea of health as wealth, riches. This age-old idea is linked to the traditional economy and is the expression of rural society where life is possible only by daily toil, as proverbs analysed by F. Loux show. Holding health in high esteem does not mean considering it as an end in itself but rather as one of the prerequisites of life which finds its meaning in work and activity. This health is inherited at birth and is the only wealth that can be bestowed, which makes childhood a time of special privileges. This heritage must be looked after to prevent it from diminishing and deteriorating over time. To a certain extent, this implies equipping themselves with the means of preventing, or at least delaying the inevitable wearing down of health, so as to be able to face up to the demands of everyday life and to cope with the stress of work. It could be asked whether the theory of human capital (with respect to health) is not based on this traditional concept of health. According to this theory, health can be considered as a durable good of which each person receives a certain amount at birth. It is subject to depreciation over the years but can be renewed by an opportune "investment" in a combination of "health production" factors, such as medical care or preventive measures.[29]

If being healthy is this group's main aim, it may seem paradoxical that they do not spare too much thought for their eating habits. In fact, they hardly ever class food and eating habits among the elements contributing to a healthy life and little mention is made of food production methods or even diet composition. These people do not complain of overeating or unhealthy eating. However, bitter remarks about neighbouring families who are "accused" of undernutrition and even malnutrition show how their interest in children's welfare extends to their food. It is important to eat well, that is, to eat enough and regularly, as can be seen in the importance this group says that it gives to the number of calories and to mealtimes. This view of the diet calls to mind the results of C. & C. Grignon's study on common tastes.[30] This preoccupation with quantity and regularity seems to derive its meaning from the two elements which are essential to this health type: children and work. Right from childhood, one of the main constituents of a healthy base, is sufficient food to insure bodily growth. A strong, resistant body, ready to meet the demands of work. From a very early age, children should also acquire a certain regularity in their way of life as regards sleeping, mealtimes and cleanliness. This is because all habits are organized with what gives a meaning to life, work, in mind. The body must be fostered so physical activity and sport are considered "instrumental" by the urban lower classes even though they do not act accordingly. As for the farmers, the very idea of physical exercise makes them smile: their work is, by definition, physical exercise, and their body is their main tool. They are also the only ones who speak of various habits as of one whole, and of the body, nature and society as a harmonious entity. The type of food, the amount of sleep, depend on the work rhythm, which in turn depends on the season.

Although it is work that gives this health type its meaning, little is said about it. It is ever-present but never elaborated on. Being healthy means being able to work, work is a criterion for good health and health is an indicator of the capacity to participate in the working world because the healthy person can do anything, even build his own house, according to a worker in the Paris region. Although the answers to the questionnaire clearly reveal that these people have the longest working hours (three out of four work 40 hours a week or more) and that they are the ones who most frequently declare their work is not very enriching, they do not talk about their professional life and its constraints nor even about working conditions. There is no talk of work as an "experience" but of work as a "necessity" because one must work to live. They have nothing to say on the matter because there is nothing to be said, but being able to work means everything is alright. Work is a point of reference to which a moral endurance and duty is more or less attached. Work dictates and organizes life and must be continually affronted. Consequently, there is not much time left for moping and thinking "too much" about oneself. Anyhow that is a good thing because too much moping "softens people" and they fall ill. It is important to be in control of oneself and assume one's responsibilities. However, when illness does occur, it upsets the points of reference and causes many problems even if it takes time to recognize and accept it. They talk a great deal about illness and illnesses, especially those connected to activity and work because working also exposes people to illness. In fact, one out of two people talks of heart problems associated with overwork and also of fatigue and of various aches and pains. This is the only group where mention is made of handicaps (deafness, bad eyesight) and occupational illnesses. Illness is always associated with activity and daily life because it prevents them from doing, working, acting, and for three out of four people, this is what gives it its meaning. It is therefore logical that the causes to which this group attributes illness are mainly bad living and working conditions. As regards the attention they give to children, they lay special emphasis on sentimental and personal problems as being at the root of certain illnesses. It will be noted that farmers talk of "healthy fatigue" with respect to their work, comparing it with office and factory work which causes nervous fatigue. Thus illness is a cause of concern in that it upsets daily life and by preventing work, can lead to marginalization. Nonetheless, this does not lead them to have frequent recourse to preventive health care. They only consult a doctor as a last resort because the endurance and work ethic is strongest in these categories for whom a visit to the doctor implies both a financial and psychological cost. So when they talk about health care it is above all in terms of equipment and cost. They consider social security to be a social progress but one that has not managed to attain its goal of completely eliminating inequality and which has been somewhat distorted because of abuses.

In this category, health as capital is the reference value, the only wealth they can give to their children, and the only wealth they possess and which allows them to work. Life centres around children and work and they are what give the different physical and social habits their meaning. The elements of the endurance and duty ethic noted here illustrate the meaning that the lower classes, represented in this health type, give to their lives.

Health depends on ...

There is a way of looking at health that is expressed by only two people in ten in urban areas. They see health as a product which can be more or less controlled. In the "health product" type, health is understood as the result of a set of various and varied factors, such as housing, sleep, work and medicine.... Health is the product of personal behaviour, living conditions, and the social system. For this group, "health-product" is a personal value, a supreme reference to which everyone submits his life. All habits are organized around it and are a constant negotiation between what can be controlled and what cannot, between private and public life, between pleasure and risk. In the last resort, health becomes the very definition of life itself, according to I.K. Zola. The sociological composition of this type is mainly Parisian, over forty, from middle-to-high income households. Should this be taken to mean that health begins to worry those who are over forty in certain social classes? To a certain extent, this idea of health as a value reflects the questioning prevailing in the medical field today. However, the redefinition of values is not just the work of those in the profession but is part of a social logic involving wider socio-economic interests, interests which perhaps could be expressed by the social classes in this health type which (in Pierre Bourdieu's words) we could call "la petite bourgeoisie nouvelle".[31]

The way in which those in this category express themselves is one of the elements which help to give its meaning to their concept of health: a discourse in the first person singular, emphasizing personal experiences on which they base their different habits. They focus on the "ego", which Richard Sennett[32] analyzes as follows: "the ego no longer refers to the agent or the 'doer' but to man considered as a being full of intentions and possibilities. It is of no matter what he does but only what he feels while he's doing it." This leads to the "tyrannies of intimacy". "When a society mobilizes narcissistic energies, it provides individuals with a principal totally contrary to that of a game. In this type of society, it is completely normal for artifice and convention to appear suspect. The logic behind this culture is the destruction of these two dimensions of human existence. It does so under the pretext of eliminating barriers that separate men, but it can only be done by psychologizing all the relationships of domination at work in society." Intimacy is both "a vision of social relationships and a necessity," that R. Sennett associates with the appearance of the "middle classes," with the development of technology in the tertiary sector.

All those for whom health is a product (and an output) talk about themselves and relate everything to themselves all the more willingly since they have a relatively voluntaristic conception of their daily habits and practices. This does not imply that they ignore the social aspect, quite to the contrary. However, they consider the social aspect above all as a constraint rather than a relationship. They devote themselves especially to criticizing the social model's system of norms and values, as something which is imposed on them and stifles their freedom. The model is criticized in the name of pleasure as can be seen from the attention paid to physical practices. It is in the "health-product" type that corporeal practices, whether they are eating, drinking alcohol, smoking tobacco or taking physical exercise, are held in highest esteem. They attribute great importance to appearance, form and taste. For example, eating habits are almost entirely based on food that is natural, good for your health and pleasing, as confirmed by the amount of time that they say they usually spend on preparing meals or shopping for natural, fresh produce. The notion of diet is most often associated with putting on weight and aesthetic concerns than with medical constraints. The purpose of physical exercise is to keep fit and relax. As regards smoking and drinking, this category is particularly responsive to the medical discourse on the risks involved, which they widely adopt but using different arguments. They see tobacco and alcohol as part of a way of life characterized by discontent and as the symbols of a society which exudes anxiety, smoking and drinking being remedies, immediate remedies which relax and even afford a certain pleasure. For the "health-product" social categories, physical habits are usually associated with personal pleasure but their high regard for health leads them to strike a balance between immediate pleasure and health risks. Their habits seem to obey what Pierre Bourdieu [33] calls "the duty to enjoy oneself" ethic. "This considers as a failure, and one serious enough to threaten one's self esteem, the inability to have fun, or as people love saying today with a slight thrill, "make whoopee". This is because pleasure is not only allowed, it is demanded for reasons which claim to be scientific rather than ethical. The fear of not having enough pleasure, the logical consequence of the desire to overcome the fear of pleasure, is combined with trying to discover own's own identity and body (bodily expression); relating to others or even total preoccupation with others (not considered as a group but as subjectivities trying to discover their identity), to replace an individual ethic with a cult of "personal health" and a "psychological therapy". As a perfect antithesis to "politicization", which depersonalizes personal experiences by considering them as particular cases of generic experiences common to a class, "moralization" and "psychologization" personalize experiences and are thus perfectly in harmony with the more or less secularized ways of seeking religious salvation."

However, this group's "duty of enjoying oneself" ethic and personal health cult refers back to their concern with managing or at least staying in control of life. This can be seen in the case of bodily pleasures, which are mainly a result of personal choice, as if they were based on terms of probability and as though behaviour were determined by a comparative evaluation of risk and pleasure. On the other hand, social habits, over which they have little control, are governed not by personal judgment but by socio-political rules. Work is an example of this. Caught up in a social system imposed on them, the people in this category describe a social situation and present a picture of daily life governed by work, but they do not talk about their professional lives or work experience. They simply talk about Work, the work of others and describe a situation onto which they can project their own cares: the lack of time. Time to be spent or time for consuming but which allows them to simply "be". They

consider Work, an abstract entity, as a constraint and not a social relationship lived daily, like those in the "health-illness" type. In the "health-
product" type, the basic problems do not seem to stem from the system
of production itself but rather from its relation to consumption. It is as
though work prevented them from consuming, since their main com-
plaint is that there is little time left for learning, amusement, relaxation,
family life.... Personal fulfilment through consumption, where the individual feels he can be himself, is seen to be totally independent of work
fulfilment. Nonetheless, work is also described as a risk which threatens
the individual's health and the family structure. This risk comes from
the build-up of activities (work outside the home, commuting, work in
the home) and from the very nature of the work which is not always a
choice and is not always fulfilling. The result can be depression and
"nervous disorders". So there is some criticism of the system of production but always in terms of health risks. This does not lead, however, to
thoughts of reorganizing work itself so as to give greater job satisfaction
and encourage personal fulfilment. On the contrary, this category is the
only one to suggest that the solution can be found in the sphere of
consumption. They respond to "work-constraint" and "work-risk" with
a reorganization and reduction of working hours whereby more free
time will solve the problem of a lack of job satisfaction, creativity and
initiative. This reorganization and solution-finding is not to be carried
out on an individual level but by regulations and socio-political intervention. It is a strange paradox that this very category of people who are
looking for their identity by exalting the ego, pleasure and individual
freedom, are starting to want the State to intervene to regulate and
manage their lives. Other social constraints for the personal health cult
are the pace of life, bad housing conditions, etc., a set of health risks that
are all equally responsible for today's ills, for stress, aggressiveness,
nervous tension, all lumped under the name of "nervous disorders".
Following a logic similar to that used when personal control is no longer
possible, they turn to consumption, to medical consumption, of course,
but preventive rather than curative. Prevention is given priority as a
means of informing and educating people about the risks of bad living
conditions. It is as though these groups consider that informing people
is enough to make them change their way of life and adopt a rational
behaviour. Is this attitude not characteristic of certain social classes, as
Luc Boltanski's studies revealed?[34] These classes figure in the "health-
product" type. Another of the contradictions of a class caught between
the desire to be themselves and to be in control of their lives?

For this health type, all bodily and social habits, both individual and collective, are based on the personal health cult. And if health tends to become life itself, these classes are caught in a web of contradictions, making their search for identity difficult: the ego cult as opposed to the rational management of life; the feeling of being and existing in the sphere of consumption as against the system of production's social constraints; the high esteem for individual freedom contrasted with the demand for social guarantees.

Health, hospitals, nurseries?

A minority of those interviewed see health through the social and health structure and the medical institution. In the "health-institution" type, health is considered to be a collective heritage for which society is responsible. This view is based on the idea of collective care, organized around a health care policy. As for its sociological composition, it is relatively homogeneous, composed mainly of people from middle and top management, rather young and with university degrees. Their social position clearly allows them to back up their point of view. They never talk about themselves or what they do but speak as a school headmaster, a paramedical employee or a gym teacher because their job means that they "know what they are talking about". Autonomy and personal initiative is hardly their chief worry. On the contrary, they seem perfectly aware of being caught in an overall social system that dominates them. The "each man for himself" principle and spontaneous, individual efforts are of little or no use. It could even be said that individuals are not responsible and in the end it is up to public authorities, be it the State or local bodies, to act. However, individuals acting as a group can some- times successfully bring pressure to bear on the political authorities and make them assume their responsibilities.

Beginning with health, these classes are led to consider themselves part of a comprehensive social system, where health care policy occupies an important place. Health is a largely political notion in so far as it concerns the whole society because its structures are collective and are in the hands of public authorities. All the habits of the group are based on this view of health. Specific experiences are rarely mentioned and individual bodily habits are of little interest to this category where we find the highest proportion of smokers and drinkers. Habits are only mentioned when they are part of a particular policy such as an education policy which directs or even obliges the individual, such as sports. Held

in high esteem by these classes, sport is not so much a leisure activity, a
source of enjoyment or a means of keeping fit, as an obligatory effort and
an indispensable element of a disciplined life, which should be adopted
by everybody once they have been encouraged or even forced to do so.
Sport is seen by this category as a means for introducing a policy of
encouragement either by providing a sufficient infrastructure or by
using schools as a springboard. Discipline based on collective habits is
to be encouraged and may even justify the use of force. Associations,
schools and the family should all introduce the basic principles of such
a discipline. A framework is essential especially as it is in childhood that
habits are first formed. The central privileged position of childhood can
be explained by the characteristics of this category composed mainly of
young parents mostly engaged in education. Although the "health-instrument" type sees childhood as a time of privilege because this is when
that indispensable capital, health, is constituted, this category is more
concerned with children as people to be trained and educated. Furthermore, this education is more oriented towards transmitting a system of
values and norms than constituting a "health capital" for work purposes.
Finally, collective structures and equipment guarantee that some social
questions are taken care of at a political level: health, education, leisure,
etc., call for hospitals, dispensaries, nurseries, schools, stadiums, and so
forth. This category reduces social problems to a question of resources
and institutionalizes them, and considering quantity more important
than quality. It was with this in mind that the Centre d'Etudes, de
Recherches et de Formation Institutionnelles began research on normali-
zation through collective installations.[35] For a deeper, theoretical study
of the notion of "programming", one could consider what Alain Touraine
calls, in a different context, "the programmed society".[36]

These categories hardly ever talk about their actual work experiences
or their professional lives. It is to the extent that it is part of a comprehensive social system that the problem is looked at from a specific angle,
that of town and country planning. Paradoxically, they are very critical
of a form of social organization that plans urban areas by squeezing
people into large apartment blocks far from the city centre and lacking
the necessary infrastructure of jobs, transport, and social and cultural
amenities. This segregative policy means long tiring journeys to find
work and threatens the family structure. This is especially true because
it is mainly women who are in this situation so there are repercussions
on family life, the couple and the children. The family disintegrates,
children are left to their own devices: the family no longer seems able to
assure its role of educator and guide. It can be seen that by trying to

"speak down" from their social position about others, these classes end up by being contradictory. They end up criticizing the very thing that they suggest, that is, planning and supervision, because they themselves admit that too much planning causes disintegration. They nevertheless proceed with their ideas of programming and supervising. Although they value medical institutions as places which produce scientific knowledge and progress, they nonetheless criticize a health care policy whose organization perpetuates social inequality by failing to encourage access to amenities. Lastly, all social and cultural, sports and health amenities are associated with health, the collective patrimony, of which the public authorities remain the guarantor. There is another contradiction between their words and their stated habits. While they emphasize the importance of collective amenities, all those who declared their adhesion to the "health-institution" concept admitted to consulting private physicians. This can be interpreted in the light of the transformations noted by Francis Fagnani.[37] The doctor is seen more and more as a technician, an "expert", because he no longer practices as a solitary worker but as part of a health care system: "people these days turn more to an institution than to an individual and the predominant image of doctors is changing from that of an independent worker to that of member of a collective service.... These multiple changes in the doctor's image are coherent with the increasing reputation of hospitals as seats of high technology medicine linked to the research and teaching worlds." These categories extend their desire for institutionalization to all types of medicine be it Chinese medicine, homeopathy or other "natural medicines", which they want to see regulated and incorporated into the official realm of medicine. Lastly, prevention, which is especially important for children, is often in the form of mother and child health care and school medicine is usually taken to mean compulsory preventive medicine and social security cover. This category sees prevention as the use of services and institutions rather than a change in individual behaviour and lifestyle.

In this type, where health is a direct means of access to the social organization, attention is focused mainly on State intervention which guarantees that social problems will be taken care of by collective services. Health is a collective patrimony, managed by the different institutions. For this group, programmed, planned, life is subjected to a certain discipline which may even be obligatory, especially for children. They use their social standing to lend weight to their opinions and even to give advice, but their behaviour does not exactly correspond to what they say.

Conclusion

This analysis of the emergence of the health-value in the medical field and in society in general, has helped to illustrate the meaning given by the various social actors to their acts. A shift in priorities and a redefinition of values are translated in the medical sphere by a change of object. Taking its place alongside curative and technical scientific medicine, is a more prevention-oriented type of medicine which emphasizes the risks of illness and makes the individual responsible. "Health" is taking over from "illness". In fact, medicine acquired its legitimacy on the basis of illness originating in the body. That made it necessary to develop a medical infrastructure and make treatment more accessible because what mattered most was being treated and recovering. Health, then, was the justification for the different steps taken by curative medicine. Recent years have seen a new conception of health for a number of reasons (the increasing cost of treatment, more knowledge about and new approaches to illness, criticism of the medical system, etc.) It is becoming a core concept as a result of "risk factors" identified in the individual's behaviour and the socio-economic environment. The aim is no longer to cure but to prevent; the "right to health" is being replaced by an "obligation to be healthy". Medicine's object is no longer merely illness but also health. So it is a new real life distinction between what should come under medical supervision and what should not, that is being drawn. Health is no longer the justification for medical science but the latter holds the meaning to life since we could even go so far as to say that health is life.

To the extent that values are never redefined by the profession alone, but are part of a broader socio-political logic, it seemed necessary to examine where people situate themselves in society in relation to the dividing line imposed by medical science as a natural one. The notion of health was seen as a key to the system of interpretation, beliefs and values of the different social classes. The present analysis relies on a typology drawn up on the basis of the opinions on health of a random sample of 100 people. Four "forms" of health have been distinguished, each a coherent whole based on a logic which reveals the meaning that the different categories give to their lives. In the "health-illness" form, it is illness that has a meaning. Excesses-illness, this type becomes aware of a norm through the experience of transgression and returning to equilibrium. The relationship between normality and pathology structures their discourse and dictates their habits, which are usually an integral part of the social system. They respect the "right measure" where concern about the order of things is based on the notion of life cycles and natural rhythms. The "health-instrument" form takes as its reference value, health as a capital. Children and work are the two elements around which life revolves and which give a meaning to the different physical and social habits. The lower classes which develop this form stress the endurance and duty ethic. The "health-product" type centres life around a personal health cult. For the classes in this type, the search for identity involves a series of contradictions which means they must constantly compromise between pleasure and risk, personal freedom and social conventions, the "ego" cult and a rational management of life. The "health-institutions" type conceives health as a direct means of access to social organization. All habits are seen in socio-political terms of society's taking charge, and of constraints. The social standing of these classes lends weight to their opinions but they do not always practice what they preach.

This first approach shows how different visions of reality grow up around the notion of health. In other words, health and illness are part of comprehensive systems of interpretation which allow people to situate themselves in society. While some consider illness as having a meaning, others consider health to be the signifier *par excellence*. In "instrument" and "produce" types, health appears as a personal value incorporated into a life ethic. In the "illness" type, it represents the norm and in the "institutions" type, it is directly political. Concern for quantity is overriding in "instrument" and "institution" whereas emphasis is on quality in "illness" and "product". Time is largely a social concept in "illness" and "instrument". "Product" and "institution" are mainly concerned with management and programming. Underlying these preoccupations can be noted a wider conception of the relationship between the sphere of production and that of consumption. While habits depend on the system of production in "health-illness" and "health-instrument", their meaning is given by consumption in the "health-product" and "health-institution" forms which are the experience of the better-off classes.

The following are the most significant extracts from four interviews, each an example of one of the health types.

Health-illness

Mrs. F., 48 years old, 6 children, cleaning lady. Husband: works in a mirror factory, Paris XIIth arrondissement.

"Health means being healthy and not too often ill, that's all. Anyway, I don't mope around, I don't have the time and even when things are not alright I say they are. That's the best way to stay healthy because if you pay too much heed to your body and start saying "I'm not feeling great today, I think I have to lie down", then you will be ill. Whereas if you say "O.K. so I'm not feeling great, but I'm going to get on with my business as though I were..." It's true that that perhaps only works up to a certain point. But to stay in bed, I've got to be very sick because I don't like staying in bed. I'm used to getting up at 5.30 every morning, including Saturdays and Sundays... I have six children who are always in good health. They've had measles, whooping cough and chicken pox, like all kids, but otherwise nothing. Six children take it out of you, you know, especially as I breast-fed them all. I am old-fashioned in those things; animals feed their young, mothers' milk must be better than bottle feeding. As for work, I could never work indoors, in an office where there's no air, no, that's not for me. I always leave the window ajar, even at night, it's one of my habits, but it's still not like the country, the air is not as pure. The doctor has always said that for my asthma, I should go to the country, so... I think I was born with asthma, though I don't think it'll go away like that, it'll go with me.....
Anyway, with my gang of kids, I don't have much time to think of myself, I work. "Work is healthy" that's my motto. That's the way I was brought up and I try and bring my children up not to be lazy because sometimes when there's no work, young people can get up to all sorts of things, they hang around or get into bad company. So what's important is to work, to eat moderately, be even-tempered and be there when the children need you.

I've got to be really sick before I go to the doctor's. I went when I was pregnant because I had to, and of course with the kids whenever they have a fever. A headache has to get really bad before I'll take a pill, it generally goes away on it's own. When I was young, I sometimes had headaches for a whole week, day and night, I still took nothing. Medicine cures one thing, but sets off another..... so prevention is better than cure. But if we could foresee everything, we would never be ill. If we could foresee that at such a place we would be in a draught and catch 'flu, we wouldn't go. When I was young, I had a friend who had had all his vaccinations and his parents had him vaccinated against polio, he never went to the swimming pool, but all the same, he died of polio. It's like car accidents, if you could foresee one, you wouldn't take the car out. They are unforeseeable events, we can do nothing about them or in any case, we can't foresee illness. Today perhaps more so than in the old days, but there are still certain things you can't foresee because if we could, we wouldn't wait for them to happen. Perhaps there are some things that can be foreseen: I'm not a magician or a fortune-teller, but it is normal that in this day and age, we're no longer in 1900, some illnesses can be foreseen, but concer, I don't think it can be foreseen; you only see cancer once you have it, then you try and cure it."

Health-instrument

M.S., 48 years old, welder. Wife: bank employee. Val d'Yerres.
    "For me, health is everything, if you haven't got your health, you can't work, you're held back in everything, you can't make plans, nothing, you can't go very far. For example, if you study, when your health is bad you don't have the energy to study. For manual work, it's the same, you need energy: if you have to stop constantly, it's demoralising and discourages you. You let yourself go and, as they say, you get old before your time. Today life is hard, it's rather difficult, a daily struggle. To struggle every day, you must be in good health to face up to everything, and the cost of living has become so high that you can't go overboard or buy extras, you have only yourself to count on. Nobody believes in anything anymore, neither family, religion, honesty, nor justice, everybody is wary of the next person, that's not normal for me. The harder life becomes, the more divided we are: that's not the answer. It's money that's the trouble, I believe it divides many people. The basic problem is that people do things only if they can get something out of it. It's human to want more, to get ahead, but it's the means used to achieve it that aren't: walking on everybody and everything to achieve the result. If you're not in good health, you can't work or make plans, you're at everybody's mercy, always begging aid at the town hall or wherever. But you have your pride, it's rough having to say thanks, go on your knees, complain to Peter and Paul, when you're of working age, it's lousy. But this is no longer the same problem: the illness today is work, nobody likes working. When you mention going to work, people wince. It's another mentality, a shift, an inexplicable phenomenon of modern life. That creates a new type of illness: work allergy..... There is so much waste, fruit is flung into the sea, while there are needy people who fall ill for want of food. Prevention begins at birth, or even before, in the mother. She must be ready and able to conceive a normal child, that will be to the child's credit in later life. It must start with the mother right

from the beginning: no alcohol or cigarette abuse, they are bad for the child's health. And, of course, you must keep an eye on the child, see he eats properly, has all his vaccinations. When you bring him up in good health, he is less often ill later on and you spend less on the doctor. And then there's education, they need a proper education oriented towards safeguarding the health capital, knowing what health is and not damaging it. Health is a capital, it is essential, it is a factor for success, a sound staring point. Because it is the child who suffers the consequences of being constantly ill and who has problems if he is not properly watched over or his mother did not look after herself.

Health-product

Mrs C., 41 years old, one child, director's personal secretary. Husband: accountant. Paris XIIth arrondissement.

"Health, for me is... we could talk about pollution and all that jazz... it's a health factor after all, because constant changing means working with new people, in new places. Otherwise, health problems are linked to daily life, which is no laughing matter, because working hours are exhausting, then there's commuting and coming home worn-out. It's a two-job life, all the domestic chores, that affects your health. I worry about my health when I flounder. I break down and then things go badly. O.K., I say to myself, the only solution is to work half-time. I can't change my working conditions but my job together with work at home, is too much. I think there is one way for people to feel better, by working less. We must realize that most people haven't got a highly motivated job. I have a job where I spend a third of my time doing things that interest me, and the rest of the time I do things which bore and, consequently, tire me. And then we have friends, we like to see them, so we stay up later than usual and are exhausted the next day, and so on. So we hesitate to stay up until one or two in the morning, because the next day we've got to work, it's crazy! It's a life where there's no more time for pleasure. There are health jokes: people are funny, no drinking, no smoking, no nothing, but they end up smoking to calm their nerves, drinking when they're a bit down, and so it's a vicious circle. I know that the more tired I am, the more I smoke; the more fed up I am, the more I drink, and I don't think I'm the only one, most people react like me. I think it's completely crazy to say to people: "smoke less". It would be better to say to them: "work less", but that we would never say. From time to time, I get a hold on myself, I go on a biological and health food kick, and also because it's better. When I buy bread in a health-food shop, I find it better than the disgusting loaf I buy from the local baker's. It's also a matter of taste. There are times when I say to myself: and what if I ate better", because at midday, at work, I eat a sandwich, and say to myself: "this evening I'll eat properly". At one time, I even started buying biological meat, but I had the impression that I was being ripped off. I paid much more and needed more time to shop, but I wasn't sure that it was better. It's a craze like any other. But at home we eat plain food, it's not exactly food that's bad for your health, but, now and then, I take more care, for the sake of my son and husband who tends to put on weight, rather than for my own sake, as I have no health problems. I know a particular category of people that I don't like and who are into macro-biotic food, weighing what they eat and also their feelings for others. They weigh everything, that bugs me. I say "what's the point?" I don't want to be like them, I prefer being exhausted, with my cigarettes and my normal food. Are they any the better for it? They will perhaps live a long life, it's sure they do nothing, but what a life!"

Health-institutions

M.D., 43 years old, two children, school headmaster. Wife: primary school teacher. Val d'Yerres.

"If I use the same criterion as East Germany did in its recovery plan, for them health was sports, it covered sports. For me, health is hygiene and health in all areas, i.e. permanent health check-ups, medical check-ups, sports and even a way of life, which in my opinion has also a lot to do with health. So health monitoring in schools should be much more stringent. That's where children start, action must start in schools. Today we have, I believe, one doctor for roughly three thousand kids, that's highly insufficient and, in my opinion, prevention in children is not efficient. They are more or less measured and weighed, which for me is a slapdash effort and, anyway, as it's not for all classes, not all the children go through it systematically every year. There are two compulsory check-ups, at six and at ten years of age, but in between we do the best we can; there just aren't enough doctors. The doctor who does come is a sort of factory doctor, there is no prevention. There is no preventive medicine whatsoever for National Education employees, not like some companies, where there are blood tests and follow-up. We have no health monitoring. As far as the general population is concerned, people who do sports should have medical check-ups and for that there should be sports medicine centres. When I first arrived in this school, we had, if I'm not mistaken, three doctors, now there are seven, eight, nine or ten. Some are battling to have sports medicine centres set up, there is a project for such a centre, we'll see. As for hygiene,: at one time there was a head-lice problem. That's also part of health, it's all a part of education, we have to inform parents. Health also means a proper diet. One third of the children eat at the canteen, that's the result of the crazy life their parents lead. They work in Paris, they have no time, so the children eat at the canteen. Sports are very important, by doing sports one stays healthy. It's all the craze, isn't it? In school, it's more or less compulsory, but do all children really participate? So, good health in children means a healthy diet, fresh air, sports; for adults, it means giving up smoking. Because of my job, I can do a lot. If I see a child in poor health, I warn his parents, but if they do nothing, I can call in the social services, or even the Departmental Health and Social Authorities (DDASS), who can then take much more effective action with parents and children. I insist strongly on compulsory vaccinations, and I did so in the case of BCG. This is a compulsory vaccination, but we realized that children were not being vaccinated. So, I campaigned very energetically among parents. Prevention does not merely mean preventing illnesses, it also means bringing up a child from childhood to adulthood, so that he doesn't need any medical treatment. Prevention means promoting harmonious growth in children."

NOTES

1. Claudine Herzlich, *Communication au Colloque sur la santé publique*, organized by the Institut national de la santé et de la recherche médicale (INSERM) on 8 and 9 October 1981, published by Editions de l'INSERM,1982, p. 332.
2. Jean Clavreul, *L'Ordre médical*, Paris, Le Seuil, 1977, p. 58.
3. Georges Canguilhem, *Le normal et le pathologique*, Paris, Presses universitaires de France, 1966 (2nd ed. 1972).
4. Michel Foucault, *Naissance de la clinique: une archéologie du regard médical*, Paris, Presses universitaires de France, 1963 (2nd ed. 1972. Transl.: *The Birth of the Clinic: an Archeology of Medical Perception*, New York, Pantheon, 1973).
5. Roger-Henri Guerrand, *Les origines du logement social en France*, Paris, Editions ouvrieres, 1967, p. 28.
6. Quoted by R.-H. Guerrand, *ibid.*, p.262.
7. Jacques Leonard, *La France médicale au XIXe siècle*, Paris, Julliard, coll. "Archives", 1978.

8. Quoted by J. Leonard, *ibid.*, p. 204.
9. V. Navarro, "The industrialization of fetichism: a critique of Ivan Illich", *International Journal of Health Services*, V, 1975.
10. I. Illich, *Medical Nemesis, The expropriation of health*, Calders and Boyars, 1975; R.J. Carlson, *The End of Medicine*, New York, John Wiley, 1975; J. Powles, "On the limitations of modern medicine", *Science, Medicine and Man*, I, 1973, p. 1-30; A. Cochrane, *Effectiveness and Efficiency: Random Reflections on Health Services*, London, The Nuffield Provincial Hospitals Trust, 1971.
11. Mimeo report of the Commissariat au Plan (Commission on health and health insurance, VII Plan), Paris, March 1976. Reprinted in *L'Hôpital à Paris*, March-April 1976, p. 113-159.
12. Marc Lalonde, *A New Perspective on the Health of Canadians*, Government of Canada, Ottawa, April, 1976, French-English bilingual report.
13. Report of the VII Plan, op. cit.
14. V. Fuchs, "Health care and the United States economic system", Milbank Memorial Fund Quarterly, L, 1972 (quoted by V. Navarro, op. cit.).
15. M. Renaud, "Les réformes québécoises de la santé ou les aventures d'un Etat 'narcissique'", in *Médecine et société: les années 80*, op. cit., p. 530.
16. I.K. Zola, "Healthism and disabling medicalization", in I.Illich *et al.*, *Disabling Professions*, London, 1977.
17. G. Canguilhem, op. cit.
18. Jean Carpentier, R. Castel, J. Donzelot, *et al.*, Résistances à la médecine et démultiplication du concept de santé, Report to the Comité d'organisation des recherches appliquées sur le développement économique et social (CORDES), November, 1980.
19. R. Crawford, "You are dangerous to your health: the ideology and politics of victim-blaming", *International Journal of Health Services*, VII, 1977, p. 663-680.
20. Norbert Bensaid, *La lumière médicale: les illusions de la prévention*, Paris, Le Seuil, 1981, p. 156.
21. This research which was carried out by a team of the CNRS, the Centre de recherche sur le bien-être (CEREBE), was financed by the DGRST and the CNRS. Its successful outcome was mainly owing to the active participation of Manuela Vicente. For more detailed results, see the reports of the CEREBE, written in collaboration with Alain Letourmy in July 1980 and May 1982.
22. Marc Augé, *Théorie des pouvoirs et idéologie: étude de cas en Côte d'Ivoire*, Paris, Hermann, 1975, p. xix.
23. Claudine Herzlich, *Santé et maladie: analyse d'une représentation sociale*, Paris, Mouton, 1969. Translated: *Health and Illness: A Social Psychological Analysis*, Academic Press, 1973, new edition 1981.
24. G. Canguilhem, op. cit., p. 216.
25. Françoise Loux et Philippe Richard, *Sagesse du corps: la santé et la maladie dans les proverbes français*, Paris, Maisonneuve et Larose, 1978, p.55.
26. N. Bensaid, op. cit., p. 244.

27. Raymond Illsley, *Professional or Public Health?*, London, Nuffield Provincial Hospitals Trust, 1980, p. 50.
28. N. Bensaid, op. cit., p. 192.
29. See also: Michael Grossman, *The Demand for Health, a Theoretical and Empirical Investigation*, New York, Columbia University Press, 1972.
30. C. and C. Grignon, Consommations alimentaires et style de vie: contribution à l'étude du goût populaire (Report CNRS—Institut de la recherche agronomique, September 1980).
31. Pierre Bourdieu, *La distinction: critique sociale du jugement*, Paris, Editions de Minuit, 1979, p. 409.
32. Richard Sennett, *Les tyrannies de l'intimité*, Paris, Le Seuil, 1979, p. 200, 272, 274. (The Fall of Public Man, Alfred A. Kuoff Inc., 1974).
33. Pierre Bourdieu, op. cit., p. 424.
34. Luc Boltanski, *La découverte de la maladie. La diffusion du savoir médical*, Paris, Centre de sociologie européenne, 1968, 220 p. mimeo; *Consommation médicale et rapport au corps*, Paris, Centre de sociologie européenne, 1970, 142 p. mimeo.
35. *Recherches*, No 13, December 1973: *Généalogie du capital, 1. Les équipements du pouvoir*.
36. Alain Touraine, *Production de la société*, Paris, Le Seuil, 1973; *L'après socialisme*, Paris, Grasset, 1980.
37. Francis Fagnani, La dynamique de la médicalisation, annexe No 6 to the report on "Croissance des dépenses de santé", (Actions Thématiques Programmées du CNRS), 1977, p. 19.

Chapter 7

FROM HEALING TO SALVATION: THE NEO-RURAL APOCALYPTIC COMMUNITIES IN FRANCE

D. Léger

The contents of this chapter are based on a particular empirical study which is contained in the report on neo-rural communities of an apocalyptic type in France today. Illness and health were not among the central themes of the study, at least not at the outset. The aim of the research was basically to analyse the link between these groups' independent and geographically limited survival practices together with their catastrophic beliefs, and the fact that explicit religious interests often arise within these same groups.[1] However, during the course of the research, one thing became apparent: the importance of healing, in all the communities observed, in the process of constituting an apocalyptic conscience, linking the original catastrophic conviction with a certainty that survival is possible for individuals or small groups of people who are prepared and regenerated.

This concurs with another, more general observation which is important in sociologically identifying the secular apocalyptic movement, called the ecological apocalyptic movement, the established link between the healing of the body and the salvation of the soul, present in all religious traditions with salvation doctrines. Salvation, a total definitive peace for believers, is loosely linked to the idea of restoration of the body which culminates in the resurrection, i.e. the healing of death itself. A perfect example of this logical schema can be found in the Judeo-Christian tradition. In the Old and New Testaments, the promise of bodily resurrection is not divorced from the promise to the converted people that they will enter into a new world. All biblical texts of an apocalyptic nature (not simply what is called the "Apocalypse") make this bodily resurrection the meeting point of the first and the last creation, the climax of this renewal of all things which will take place at the end of time. The only purpose of the evangelic presentation of Jesus' healing miracles was to present this eschatological horizon and at the same time show its relevance to the present day.

This permanent feature of the Christian apocalyptic tradition (and of the Christian religion in general) highlights the extent of Christianity's ambivalent attitude towards the body. The biological body is a house of sin, but it is also the ultimate manifestation of salvation. Some branches of Christianity have developed this second dimension to the point where physical regeneration is the sign and means of spiritual salvation. A good example of this are the Adventists, a movement founded in the U.S. in the 19th century on the basis of two ideologies: the late 19th century apocalyptic speculations and social hygiene, two co-existing ideological movements whose social origins can be traced to the social and cultural crisis in the countries of Europe and North America caused by the first industrial revolution.[2]

The comparison of these two observations, the importance of illness and health in the neo-rurals' ecological apocalyptic movement, and the ever presence of body healing in the religious apocalyptic movement, led us to look closer at the place given to and the transformations suffered by the representations of the ill and/or healed body in the frequently attested transmutation of this ecologic apocalyptic movement into a specifically religious apocalyptic movement.[3] We will give only a very partial sociological perspective of this transmutation process. It will be sufficient, however, to reveal what it has in common with the concern expressed by Claudine Herzlich at the end of her contribution to this book, with updating the social implications of the "quests for meaning" which are manifest today through the various forms of opposition to medical power. In this wider perspective, it may be of interest to try to grasp the ideological and social motives underlying the anti-medical movement which are expressed in the healing by a return to nature concept, and the interest may go beyond the neo-rurals who carry the autonomous survival logic to its extreme, seeking the path to autonomy in the field of health.

I DISASTER, ILLNESS AND APOCALYPSE

The word "apocalypse" is overused in everyday language. As the collective conscience becomes more aware of the major risks facing Mankind, the distinction between the apocalypse and any type of world catastrophe (or even any tragic accident where there are many victims) becomes more blurred. At the same time, its original meaning (in Greek = unveiling, laying bare or revelation of human and divine secrets) tends to be forgotten. However, according to this very definition, the apocalyptic catastrophe is not merely an earthly calamity, but a turning point, a turn in the tide of human history, the threshold of the end of time and thus the unfolding of that which had remained hidden until the fatal crisis.

All neo-rurals and ecologists, whether part of a movement or not, and more generally all those who seek the way to a "healthier", "simpler" or more "natural" life (food, sports, etc.), weigh up the dangers and contradictions of a certain type of economic growth and question the artificiality of the type of life it implies. Thus, they become part of a widespread catastrophic conscience, more or less articulate, and widespread especially among middle class intellectuals where the feeling of having no control over social and economic reality, a feeling that itself is the subjective reflection of their ill-defined position in society, becomes a vehement denunciation of the absurd state of the world. A small number of these groups, for whom we must reserve the title of "apocalyptics", have a much more radical view of these dangers. They consider that the catastrophe looming up with its multiform symptoms will mark the end of industrial society. It will cause the dramatic but effective downfall of a civilisation based on artifice and, with one fatal blow, insure the end of urban civilisation. They do not simply present an eschatological view of the renewal of all things after the final crisis, they also draw from it principles to rationally govern their everyday lives. Their aim is to prepare for the imminent living through "Hard Times" in a practical way and first an foremost by immediately giving up habits which endanger the individual and, in their clean order, help to aggravate the general threat. According to them, it is necessary to stop eating too much and badly; to refuse anything that intoxicates the body and mind; to immediately abandon the excessive pace of urban life with its noise, pollution, rhythm, and the mindless exhaustion of work where the individual has no control whatsoever over its organisation or its ends. All the common aspects of the daily lives of those living in big cities are interpreted by the new apocalyptics as direct threats to the physical and moral health of each person and as symptoms of a fatal disease which is spreading corruption through the whole society, leading it to the brink of final disaster.

This manner of associating individual illness with a general and deep degradation of the social "body" is not new. It can even to a certain degree be traced back to the view of illness as a social ill, which has been gradually repudiated since the beginning of the 20th century by the ever-more precise biological explanations of the specific aetiology of each illness.

Neither is the use of illness as a metaphor to describe society's ills very original. What does however specifically characterise the ecological, apocalyptic groups' views, is the way they mould these two levels of representation into one coherent description of the forthcoming catastrophe. And it is, in fact, coherent. They show that the depletion and degradation of the natural heritage, which drastically changes the working conditions of an economy based on the unlimited exploitation of its natural resources are directly linked to the increase of violence worldwide. Violence is breaking out in all aspects of society, form the family cell to international relations. This ecological catastrophe associated with the pollution of the air and the seas, with the destruction of the earth, the "waste invasion", and finished off by the nuclear horror, is paralleled in a very predictable manner, by political catastrophe (war) which is becoming apparent in thousands of spots around the globe. Within a few years, "the shield of plenty" will disappear in the most industrialized countries: after unemployment and inflation, economic wounds already inflicted, there is a food shortage in store for mankind. This very black picture frequently figures city-dwellers, ravenous, pouring out into the countryside, in search of means of survival. Too bad for the weakest! This unprecedented economic catastrophe will necessarily lead to an ethical catastrophe. The collective loss of values and of solidarity and the inability to communicate, already visible in urban industrial society, are but the harbingers of a barbaric future where the only principle of social order will be brute force.

Illness is the perfect symbol of the complete destruction that will leave nothing intact. Man's body already bears the scars of widespread chaos. The recent increase in system-related illnesses, the so-called "diseases of civilisation": cardio-vascular diseases, cancer, lung and skin diseases and other diseases associated with pollution, nervous disorders caused or aggravated by the stress of urban life, etc. show that everybody is affected despite tremendous medical progress. That is because man is sick "of the world" and specific technical treatment is powerless in the face of this type of imperceptible, insidious ill that implicates each person in their own destruction. Modern civilization has a poisonous effect on the body, all nature is poisoned in particular with a poison called radioactivity. Nobody can hope to escape this poisonous cycle: with the intoxication of the earth, the seeds of mankind's destruction are sown.

"(...) They bore into you as far as they could and planted this growth in your stomach. They poisoned your vessels and arteries with an illness all the more painful because it could not be seen. An illness that the rivers bear underground to feed the springs. A white feathered seagull, a shrew cross forbidden territory and return bearers of death (...) Fog thick with poison seeps into the grass that cows graze and ruminate in their stomachs and ruddy-cheeked farmers' wives milk it from their udders and feed it to their greedy babies. Sea currents bear the poison into the flesh of yawning oysters and fat mussels, swish it through lichens and algae and fishermen's big basket-nets bring the rotten catch home....."[4]

This extract from Xavier Gauthier is an ideal and typical example of the neo-apocalyptical view of illness, seen as the individual equivalent of the general destruction of nature. From this viewpoint, illness is the individual epitome of catastrophe. According to the most pessimistic forecasts, prompted by bacteriological weapons research and studies on the prospects of increased world-wide famine (with all their biological and genetic consequences), illness can be considered as one of the most likely forms that the wholesale destruction of mankind will take.

The apocalyptics do not see illness as merely incidental, the human side-effects of the major threats known to mankind. It *is* the catastrophe, a way of punishing. If the catastrophe is nature's vengeance on a planetary scale, illness is the form taken by this "vengeance" on a personal scale.

This notion of catastrophe-as-a-means-of-punishment, leading to illness-as-a-means-of-punishment is fundamental for the development of an apocalyptic conscience. Images of this catastrophe are dominated by radiation, gulags, famine and cancer and correspond to one interpretation of the causes of the foreseeable crumbling of the foundations of our society and history. Beyond its immediate causes, the roots of the ultimate crisis lie in the boundlessness of human pride, the anthropocentrism at the basis of the Promethean illusion about man's illimited power over nature. Man considers the universe a place set aside for him, where he can give full reign to his desire for power. He has lost all sense of his own dependence on his natural environment. Or rather, he only sees it as the vestige of a former yoke that scientific and technical developments will help to throw off. The environment is no longer the womb where man is formed, it is an unessential context, a source of productive energy, a space to be exploited (in all senses of the word). The body itself is instrumentalised and is no longer considered to be above all man's link with his environment. It is only worth what it can produce or consume. But the price man pays for the illusion that he is lord and master over nature is the loss of his own identity. He has lost the sense of man and environment as one entity, which was, for Alan Watts, the only reality in life. It is no mere chance that A. Watts is quoted here. There are many obvious similarities between the American counter-culture which have survived and become what is today called, on the other side of the Atlantic, "the new spiritual culture" and the neo-rural apocalyptics who are closer to us. They are aware of the same threats and give them the same diagnosis: "We have forgotten that nature is quite simply the universal continuum of which we are an extricable part."[5]

This "forgetting" signifies our loss, set in the contradictions of a materialistic society which has become a slave to man's "needs" just when it claims to have shaken off nature's yoke.

"The end of the world", affirms T. Roszak, "was announced to St John by a heavenly voice thundering down like the sound of the great waters. But the voice which comes today exhorting us to exhaust the gloomy myth of a settling of scores are our shrill voices, chiming in the middle of casual conversation about the various ways the world might be destroyed: By the nuclear Armageddon, the disappearance of the seas, the deterioration of the atmosphere, the massacre of the innocents, imminent universal famine..... If these dreadful ills do befall us, we can not put them down to the caprice of some ill-meaning God. They are the result of an eminently practical, harsh and materialistic policy, ruled by the law of dollars and cents."

II HEALING AND RETURN TO NATURE

There is, however, one solution to this absolute chaos and that is the one which is at the heart of the ecological apocalyptics' eschatological hope. Like the American "new spirituals", they propose a return to nature and natural order as the only means of coherently reorganizing society and reestablishing an ecological balance. Regeneration can only be achieved by physically abandoning the artificial universe of urban industrial society and going to live close to nature and rediscovering the basic rules of survival; building one's own house, producing one's own food, finding oneself again by mastering one's immediate surroundings on one's own scale and "living in harmony with the ecosystem, neither cold nor hungry, co-operating with nature by using its alternative and renewable resources."[7] A certain number of groups can be found in France inspired like their fellow Americans, by oriental philosophy and mysticism, often influenced by the writings of Henri David Thoreau[8] and his experiments in "the simple life": they preach the ethic of frugality whereby one chooses to provide for all one's needs by being self-sufficient. Their aim for simplicity, a condition for real submission to the laws of nature, is mainly sought in housing and feeding themselves. Rather than isolate man from his natural environment, a house should permanently immerse him in it, reminding him that it is both benevolent and demanding. A house should be light, makeshift, mobile and adaptable, like a second skin to its dwellers. By voluntarily submerging himself in nature, man will re-develop his original sensitivity atrophied by modern life. He will re-acquire his former know-how, be a person of his own making and thus rediscover his real identity. From this point of view, the only way to salvation is by being aware of one's dependence on nature and striving to live this independence logically.

The French neo-rurals have another vision of the Apocalypse which is more specific to them. They see the return to nature as equivalent to returning to a traditional rural society of the past. They recommend reverting to age-old methods of cultivation land, reintroducing traditional crops and livestock, adopting eating habits and artisanal techniques from the past, reviving rural sociability etc. At first sight, this neo-agrarianism seems slightly archaic: it seeks to rediscover ancestral rhythms and identify with a stage of economic and social development which is long past. It is not the past for the past's sake that they seek, however, but rather the high degree of adaptation between man and his environment, which was perfected by societies faced with the problem of surviving in extremely difficult conditions. In the attempt to harmonize man's relationship with his surroundings, each community, depending on its circumstances, finds a historical reference in the nomads of Ancient Palestine, the North and South American Indians prior to colonisation, the geomantic peasants of ancient China and in particular medieval monks. The less symbolic but more down to earth examples of borrowing from local tradition as regards crops, livestock, food and medicine, marks a return to the former equilibrium between man and the land he inhabits. By fixing broken benches, reintroducing seasonal migration and cultivating abandoned land, he is stepping into the shoes of the old land-clearer and becoming a pioneer. The foundations of a new culture are thus laid. It is more appropriate to speak of "restitution" than archaism, since this underlines the role of the imagination in the search for a traditional solution to new needs created by the decline of technical industrial civilisation. For this it resorts mainly to the collective memory of a society with deep rural origins.

These two versions of the ecological apocalypse dictate very different approaches to the search for practical means of survival but neither of them gives a clear idea of their representations of illness and health nor their therapeutic practices.

One idea common to all the groups concerned is that the only road to recovery for all those who, more often than not, are "ill without knowing it", is through the reappropriation of their own body and making it dependent on its immediate surroundings. Recovery is not possible without a complete change of life, an overall putting-back-in-order that requires of each person a real conversion. It is by constantly challenging nature and reconstituting his original physical abilities, lessened or damaged by the artificiality of urban life that each person revives himself. This overall conception of recovery is linked to the mistrust these groups have in "heavy" medical technology and the extreme specialisation of its practitioners.[10] This specialisation implies a fragmentary and limited vision of the human organism which all the neo-apocalyptics, whether or not they have read Edward T. Hall's[11] writings, try and re-situate into its territorial and environmental context. The interest all these groups share in "natural" medicine, especially herbal medicine may sometimes be justified by experience acquired from traditional societies or the coherent logic of a naturalist philosophy but they all show a strong desire to resist institutionalised medicine through autonomous therapeutic know-how. It is part of a strategy to "break all links" with a doomed society and rebuild a natural order in small groups and in a limited geographical area. As one of the most representative groups pointed out "we must prove that somewhere in between the desert and the city, there are spaces where small groups of people can reforge a link with the organic form of life inhabiting those spaces."[12]

Must we conclude that illness could be absent from such places? None of the apocalyptic groups we met asserted this, although they all think that returning to a more natural life, more in line with basic biological rhythms would immediately eliminate many pathological symptoms both of a physical and psychical nature. In this context, illness would no longer be considered, as is generally the case in the dominant society, an outrageous and intolerable accident but could be lived individually and collectively as an indicator of unresolved tensions within the groups or in its relation to its territory. It would act as an alarm mechanism, reminding man of the precariousness of the equilibrium, like a "call to order".

The idea of illness as a "call to order" is fundamental to most of the neo-apocalyptic therapeutic experiments. Many groups take in anybody in distress such as drug addicts, overeaters and depressives. The hospitality they receive is generally informal and is simply determined by the group's idea of its exemplary mission and its sense of responsibility for those who are the prime victims of the madness they condemn. However, this hospitality is sometimes systemized, an invitation to join the community being proposed as a therapeutic solution. In this case no particular "treatment" is administered to the "guest" (never referred to as a "patient" to avoid a patient-healer situation arising.) He is, however, asked to give up, without a transition period or any compromising, the "bad habits" which are at the root of his ills and to adhere strictly to the group's rules regarding food, work, timetable, and sexuality. Acceptance of the community's social order, which is itself part of a highly rationalized way of managing one's surroundings, is a concrete and symbolic sign of "the lost one" returning to an ordered universe, and accepting the authority prevailing in the group which in all cases studied was the ultimate sign of this return.[13] The fact that agricultural work with its objective demands (natural cycles, seasonal recurrences) constitutes the material framework for community order, gives it a "natural" basis and hence legitimacy in the eyes of those concerned. The dividing line between order and disorder is to be found in the soil, separating the regenerated and potentially saved (even if they have not yet fully recovered from their state of total physical decrepitude) from the majority who (ill without knowing it and so with no desire to be healed) contribute to their own undoing.y

III ANTI-MEDICAL AND SOCIAL PROTESTATION

This concept of healing as a personal conversion and a complete change in lifestyle contrasts with the dominant concept of illness and treatment as a specific remedy for a specific, accidental and temporary disorder. It is not necessarily incompatible with the idea of some physicians that changes are needed in urban lifestyle if the harmony between man and his environment is to be reestablished and an "ecological view of health" developed.[14] The large majority of new apocalyptics show, however, as little confidence in this updated medical approach as they do in various examples of ecologically minded reform which simply recommend adapting the socio-economic system to a new set of data, particularly to signs of a scarcity of natural resources. Their criticism of the medical system is not merely aimed at the technical aspect of modern therapeutic methods. The established social relationship between patient and physician, and between the sick and society at large is questioned in a purportedly radical way. This social relationship of dependence puts the sick in the ambiguous position of assisted and outcast at the same time, reflecting in a quasi-paradigmatic fashion the general condition of all social "misfits", all those whose place in society is ill-defined. The type of social protest at the basis of the "back to nature" movement can be very clearly seen in the anti-medical protest taken by all neo-rurals[15] and systematically put into practice by apocalyptic groups experimenting in therapeutic autonomy.

Most neo-rurals come from the intellectual middle classes which were greatly shaken by the political and cultural events of 1968-70, and even more so by the massive unemployment of 1975-80. For most of them, communal life and going back to nature were initially a way of utopic protest with no political aims, and a reclassification strategy aimed at reducing the gap, which they found it hard to accept, between their level of culture and their social status. Some who had fled to the countryside to adopt a communal way of life through "escaping from society", had become the ideal pawns in a government strategy to repopulate desolate areas.[17] The fact that many of these groups turned apocalyptic can be explained by the relative failure of this compensatory strategy (or at least the serious difficulties it encountered). It is worth noting that the groups with the most elaborate catastrophic views today are the very groups that expressed most clearly (and often with most bitterness too) the impossibility for them to become fully integrated into rural society. They often admit to having been unaware of its contradictory nature which they attribute to "contamination" from urban, industrial society due to the economic, social, political and cultural dependence of these peripheral regions. The ecological apocalypse is the reply on an ideological level to a second-degree compensatory movement: these cultural misfits, the neo-rurals, are out of place in local relationships just as they had occupied a very uncertain place in society as "intellectual proletarians". Escaping to the country did not change the subjective or objective uncertainty of their place in society in any way. Some of them manage to make this uncertainty the basis of a definition of their local and social status. In many ways they become subsidized experimenters in what they want to be a new model of daily life. Most of them hover between two cultures and two societies (intellectual and rustic, urban and rural) where they no longer, or never have, belonged.[19]

Highly dramatizing the future is the only means they have of showing their cultural disposition for dispelling the objective and subjective difficulties they have in fitting into society, by commenting the great evolutions of humanity. Being symbolically in control of foreseeable changes (mainly the handling of ecological ideas) enables them to escape from the actual powerlessness of their situation and at the same time provides a socially acceptable form of anti-institutionalism which that situation imposes.[20] Just as they use their catastrophic vision of the future to justify the choice of autonomous communal life, they present nature as an ordered world, revealing a vision of society adapted to the hopes of a social class which occupies an uncertain, precarious and ambiguous place in society. Similarly, they often end up identifying natural order with bygone times when social behaviour responded, according to them, to the needs of the environment. The reference to order in bygone times, counterbalancing this refusal of the world such as it is, backed up by the belief that the end of the world is near, gives their communal quest for exemplary marginality a meaning. Max Weber, talking about "the flight from society of intellectuals" who are in constant deep conflict between their need for meaning, the present state of the world, and the possibility of fitting into it, indicates that it can take the form of "escaping to a nature unspoiled by human institutions" (Rousseau) or it can be a romantic escape to join "simple folk" as yet uncorrupted by human conventions (Russian *narodnischestvo*).[21] In a social and economic context where there is little hope of such radical changes in society, this "escape from the world" takes the form of a fascination with a past where groups of human beings, organized into carefully regulated groups, enjoy a harmonious relationship with nature.

Thus, applied research by the neoapocalyptics in herbal medicine, iridology, health food, etc., is simply the prolongation in a different form of the anti-institutionalism of 1968-70, when medicine, universities, the Church and political parties were part of a general refusal of the bureaucratic and repressive mentality gradually dominating society as a whole. The distinguishing mark of the apocalyptics is that they constitute their own alternative therapeutic methods and show great interest in popular knowledge (agricultural, culinary and meteorological), local culture and

religious traditions of the past. One way in which these teachers, reform-
ers, and leaders symbolically assert and question the uncertainty of their
own cultural position is by reinstating cultural aspects (popular medicine for example) that are ignored, eclipsed and shunned by the dominant technical and scientific culture. Their interest is part of a
rehabilitation of what is called a prelogical way of thinking according to
modern criteria for knowledge. It is the way for these intellectual pariahs
(as Weber would say) to "distinguish themselves from the legitimate
knowledge holders". This distinctive and compensatory function becomes even more obvious when one compares the relative importance
of parallel therapeutic research in the communities to the number of its
members belonging to the medical (often paramedical) professions or
having abandoned university studies which would have led to those
professions. The importance they all attach to becoming autonomous
may be for some a sort of revenge (explicit or implicit) on the medical
profession and its self-perpetuating and auto-selective procedures or it
may be direct compensation for a "vocation they did not follow".[22] In any
case, whatever may be the backward or archaic effects of rejecting
technical medicine for age-old medicine, it can only be understood in the
light of this utopian movement[23] which reveres a bygone age. They
revert to the resources of nature and bygone times as a way of underlin-
ing the illusion of progress which, far from assuring a brighter future,
destroys mankind's chances of having any future. Thus it can also be
seen to have a mobilizing function: cultural elements from the past
stimulate a desire for the new world which will follow the forthcoming
catastrophe.

IV FROM HEALING TO SALVATION/FROM
ECOLOGICAL APOCALYPSE TO RELIGIOUS
APOCALYPSE

The discovery that "natural medicine" (as the utopian solution proposed
by an anti-social movement of which the anti-medical movement is the
moving force) has two functions, a distinctive function and a mobilizing
function, strengthens the conclusions that could be drawn from an
analysis of the renewed interest shown by these groups in the great
religious traditions of mankind. As is the case with all traditional wisdom, that which gives religion its value in the eyes of some neo-apoca-

lyptics is the fact that it was, and continues to be, the main target of modern rationalism. Precisely because it is not in line with the dominant culture, religion can act as a reservoir of mobilizing symbols. In this light, adopting age-old medical practices and returning to religion may seem two parallel examples among others of a reaction against the modern world, all the more interesting because it is most common among intellectuals, in a social class which is neither pre-political nor pre-scientific but rather post-political and post-scientific.

The coherence of these two examples can also be seen if we look at how one can lead to the other. Looking at it from this point of view, the two are no longer parallel but rather interwoven in a sort of chain that guarantees the development of an ecological apocalyptic movement into a religious apocalyptic movement. By examining existing information three distinctive steps in the process can be seen, each one corresponding to a successive stage of integration in the community.

The first stage is when discussions about the ecological catastrophe become an actual quest for autonomous survival. Instead of simply shouting about the threats facing mankind, they begin, at this point, to experiment a way of life that will enable them to survive those difficult times, as a group and in a geographically limited area. At this stage, when they come to actually putting their words into action, nature ceases to be a mythical reference to lost harmony and becomes a test to be faced daily. If the group is to live entirely on what it manages to produce on bad land, often devastated since it had been abandoned, they must battle constantly against difficulties that they were ill prepared for. Clearing the land and carefully enriching the soil implies a rational organization of community life and intense use of labour and even then they often only manage to provide the bare essentials by strictly limiting individual and collective needs. The price of autonomy is an austere life of hard work organized around a tightly knit community which assures its members are constantly on guard and at the same time supports and strengthens their apocalyptic conviction.

The second stage is when the ethic of frugality, which always accompanies ideological references to "nature's laws", ceases to be a vague call for primitive simplicity. At this stage, the group creates the values and rules that respond to its real needs of its survival as a group. The need to establish itself on the territory, for the whole group to work towards the same objective, to manage its territory wisely and other needs are defined more precisely in ethics which replace the original vague reference to "nature". These ethics are to be found in the rules (written and unwritten) for communal living that dictate the conditions for participating in community life, sharing the workload among its members, organizing its sexual life and power sharing.

However, these rules for living "according to nature's laws and so, according to good laws" do not simply provide guidelines for solving any problems that may arise within the group itself or between the group and the outside world. They draw the dividing line which sets apart all those who have opted for "the new world". They symbolize and represent the group's separation from the world. The rules vary according to the group's relationship with the territory from which it draws its means of survival. However, they always strengthen the tendency which all groups trying to survive in difficult conditions have, to develop a "dichotomizing awareness of the world", drawn from daily experience which both gives it a meaning and a direction. The third rung on the ladder going from ecology to religion depends on the form this dichotomizing awareness takes. At this stage, the desire for a healthier, simpler, more natural and human life, which was the original response to an awareness of the threats menacing industrial society, becomes a question of salvation, implying a necessary separation between those who will be saved and those who will not. The idea of "the elect" common to this approach to salvation based on a dichotomizing awareness of the world[24] and to various religious views of salvation is the basis for their subscription to spiritual traditions which can provide them with acceptable references (namely by supplying a "host of witnesses" from all ages and places). The daily struggle for survival, against a threatening environment (be it openly hostile or barren) form the basis of a symbolic contrast between the community and the world, order and disorder, good and bad. An image of the world based on this daily experience implies a series of symbolic contrasts, taking the contrast between sacred and profane as model.

At each stage of the transformation from an ecological apocalyptic movement to a religious apocalyptic movement, the question of illness and recovery plays a central role. It is one way of relating the ideological process, schematized above in an idealistic form, to people's daily life.

At the first stage, that of "putting words and thoughts into action", the experience of illness (or memory of, or fear of such an experience) frequently acts as the trigger. It introduces a threat into people's daily lives, by embodying the risks we all face. It acts as an "alarm signal" (as often depicted in tales of religious conversion) prompting the person to turn over a new leaf by suddenly presenting him with two alternatives, one of which may be death.

At the second stage, that of "setting things in order", emphasis is placed on what is needed for recovery, justifying the efforts and endurance of all those participating in the communal quest for autonomy. They are able to bear the burden imposed by strict adherence to the Rule better, if there is a physically quantifiable improvement in their general well-being. The price may be high but the rewards are not simply the far-off promise of the new world to come. The immediate reward is a "body restored to health". The direct therapeutic effects (noted in every case) of an extremely regular life with incontestable and fundamental aims such as survival, together with the effects of psychological stability from being part of a world "free of uncertainties",[25] is a preview of what the eschatological promise will bring. The recovery of health is evidence of a new world and provides utopic confirmation. What applies to individuals applies to groups. The efforts of the many groups that welcome people in distress, although perhaps incomprehensible from a purely economic point of view, can be justified by the results hoped for and often achieved.[26] It is, however, at the third stage, which is crucial for the group's religious orientation and is the point when a dichotomizing awareness of the world develops, that the reference to illness and good health is especially important. It is part of a common framework of references in the form of a permanent, firmly established, contrast between those who are physically part of the restored order and those who continue to live a disordered life; between those who are cured and those who are ill. Insofar as it depicts the antagonism between order and disorder, this contrast resembles another contrast, the one setting the vegetable garden and the clearing apart from the thicket, the heath and barren land, which forms part of a common awareness resulting from the shared daily task of clearing the land and making it habitable.[27] It also provides a normative value: separating those who have been converted and who are now nature's allies from those who persist in the fatal belief that their body is a tool. A similar distinction will be made at the time of the catastrophe between who is to be saved and who will perish. Not only that, it is the first step in the process. The present geographical segregation of communities and society is likened to the future division of the whole of mankind. The contrast sick/healed (which has been personally experienced by all those concerned) provides the link between the descriptive contrast between order and disorder and the normative contrast between salvation and damnation. These two forms of contrast converge in the paradigmatic contrast between sacred and secular.

So if it as accepted that this view of illness and health falls within a "religious" context arising from the daily life of a group faced with the

222   THE MEANING OF ILLNESS

problem of survival on the land in difficult conditions, it can also be
noted that within this neo-religious approach, it is the idea of healing so
understood which conveys the meaning of salvation in a simple, down-
to-earth, realistic way.

NOTES

1. During this study on apocalyptic groups, over ten communities in the
   Cevennes, Southern Alps, and Pyrenees were closely and continuously
   observed for three years. Cf. B. Hervieu and D. Léger, *Des communautés pour
   les Temps Difficiles*. Néoruraux ou nouveaux moines, Paris, le Centurion,
   1983.
2. For more information on Adventism consult Brian Wilson in *Les sectes
   religieuses*, Paris, Hachette, 1970.
3. On this particular point, see D. Léger, "Apocalyptic ecologique et 'retour'
   de la religion", *Archives de sciences sociales des religions*, 53/1, 1982.
4. Xavière Gauthier, "Je te croyais indomptable...", *Silex*, No. 18-19, (special
   edition about ecological problems).
5. Théodore Roszak, *Où finit le désert?*, Paris, Stock, 1973, p. 31. Over the last
   two or three years, there have been more and more publications in French
   on what could be called the "returning awareness" of the "New Age" which
   is closely connected to this deep feeling of crisis. An example is Paule
   Salomon, *Les nouveaux aventuriers de l'esprit*, Paris, Albin Michel, 1979;
   Marilyn Ferguson, *Les Enfants du Verseau*, Paris, Calman-Levy, 1980; J.M.
   Schiff, *L'age cosmique aux USA*, Paris, Albin Michel, 1980; S. Crossman and
   E. Fenwick, *Le Nouvel Age*, Paris, Le Seuil, 1981.
6. T. Roszak, op. cit., p. 9.
7. M. Jourdan, *La Maison sur la montagne*, Paris, Editions Entente, 1980, p. 9.
8. H.D. Thoreau, *Walden ou La Vie dans les bois*, Paris, Aubier Montaigne, 1968.
   Cf. also: Michele Flack, *Thoreau ou la sagesse au service de l'action*, Paris,
   Seghers, 1973 (Mr. Flack's commentary is even more known to neo-rurals
   than Thoreau's writings themselves).
9. "A house is a garment and nothing more. As with a garment, when inside
   it, one should not feel suffocated, emprisoned or separated from the
   universe." *La Maison sur la montagne*,op. cit., p. 20-21. This "living house"
   resembling a primitive hut can, however, use the resources of the most
   advanced technology to achieve its aim of being light and open. *Vibrations
   solaires*, published in 1979 (34, 3100 Toulouse) by the Association Planetaire
   des Technologues Doux, tells of an experiment in the use of solar energy
   to insure the autonomy of a light wooden dwelling in the mid-Ariege
   mountains. Various do-it-yourself manuals such as *Manuels d'Autocon-
   struction*, published by Editions Alternative et Parallele, give a good idea
   of the technical possibilities tried out today by a certain number of "newly
   housed" and neo-rural communities.

10. Ivan Illich's book *Némésis médicale*, Paris, Le Seuil, 1975, has greatly contributed to this train of thought. It is one of the basic reference books for neo-rurals.

11. Edward T. Hall, *La dimension cachée*, Paris, Le Seuil, 1971, considers territory as an extension of the human and animal organism.

12. Charter of F... (Gard),

13. Readers will find a more detailed analysis of this aspect of the return to order in D. Léger's "Charisma, Utopia and Communal Life: The case of Neorural Apocalyptic Communes in France", *Social Compass* XXXIX/1, 1982, p. 41-58.

14. Cf. P.M. Brunetti, "Pour une notion écologique de la santé", *Silex*, No. 18-19, 1980.

15. Their protest is very radical in principle but in reality, they very often resort to classical medicine, "in emergencies or in very serious cases".

16. Cf. D. Léger and B. Hervieu, *Le Retour à la Nature: au fond de la forêt ... l'Etat*, Paris, Le Seuil, 1979.

17. This concept of compensatory strategy is borrowed from Pierre Boudieu, "Classement, declassement, reclassement", *Actes de la recherche en sciences sociales*, No. 24, 1978, p. 17: "Strategies used either for trying to avoid being "declassed" and rejoining the path of another class, or to continue the interrupted course of an aspired-to path."

18. Max Weber, *Economie et société*, Paris, Plon, 1971, p. 525.

19. It must be remembered that these are model paths, in reality, individual situations are always more complex, contradictory and irregular.

20. Pierre Bourdieu,op. cit.

21. Max Weber, op. cit., p. 524-525.

22. A large proportion of the neoapocalyptic community is from the paramedical or sociomedical profession, and of them, a large number speak of their past school and professional lives in the following terms: "What I really wanted to do was medicine, but for certain reasons (...) I could not."

23. Defining Utopia as Jean Seguy does: "A call to the past which is often seen as a magnified Golden Age, compared to the present, which is rejected, and looking towards a radically different future." ("Une sociologie des societes imagines: monachisme et utopies", *Annales E.S.C.*, XXVI, 1971, p. 328-354.)

24. All known religious beliefs, be they simple or complex, have one common feature: "They imply a classification of those things, both real and imaginary, that are important to man, into two groups, two contrasting types, generally given two distinct names which signify sacred and profane. The twofold division including on the one hand that which is sacred and on the other that which is profane, is the characteristic feature of religious thinking." (Emile Durkheim, *Les Formes élémentaires de la vie religieuse*, 5th ed., Paris, Presses universitaires de France, 1968, p. 50-51.)

25. This lack of incertitude is due above all to an exhaustive and rhythmic use of time which liken these communities to the monastic model.

26. We were able to observe directly the remarkable efficacy, often certified by doctors, of these methods of personal restructuration practised by a certain number of these groups.

27. This biblical image of the garden (Paradise found) contrasted with the forest is a common metaphor for spiritual life "the victory of order over disorder". (Cf. Les Sermons de Saint Bernard.) On this subject, see: G. Duby, *Saint Bernard, L'art cistercien*, Paris, Flammarion, 1979, p. 112-113.

28. Here meant in a non-specifically religious sense: having changed their lives radically.

Index

For Product Safety Concerns and Information please contact our
EU representative GPSR@taylorandfrancis.com Taylor & Francis
Verlag GmbH, Kaufingerstraße 24, 80331 München, Germany